Contents

ISLER'S POCKET DICTIONARY OF DIAGNOSTIC TESTS, PROCEDURES & TERMS

Charlotte Isler, R.N.

Medical Economics Company
Book Division
Oradell, New Jersey 07649

Library of Congress Cataloging in Publication Data

Isler, Charlotte.
Isler's pocket dictionary of diagnostic tests, procedures & terms.

Bibliography: p.
1. Diagnosis—Dictionaries. 2. Diagnosis, Laboratory-Dictionaries. I. Title. II. Title: Pocket dictionary of diagnostic tests, procedures & terms.

RC71.I83 616.07'5 80-20157
ISBN 0-87489-189-2 (pbk.)

Design by JoAnne Cassella

ISBN 0-87489-189-2

Medical Economics Company
Oradell, New Jersey 07649

Printed in the United States of America

Preface

As a health worker, you've seen it many times: A patient who's just been told that he needs one or more tests, or maybe a more complex diagnostic procedure, is full of apprehension and probably remembers only part of the doctor's explanation. He's worried about his health, about how the tests will be done, and what they're going to show.

You're sympathetic to the patient's fears, and you'd like to reassure him by explaining once more what's going to happen. But lab tests may not be part of your work, and so you may be just as puzzled as the patient by lengthy laboratory terms, or worse, abbreviations that are meaningless to both you and the patient.

Anyone who is going to be tested has a right to know what the test is, why it's being done, and what it's likely to show. This book takes the mystery out of the world of lab tests and diagnostic procedures most commonly performed in hospitals, nursing homes, doctors' offices, and other health facilities. Here you'll find all the tests, terms, and diagnostic procedures you want to know, or that a patient may ask you about. You can easily consult this guide, or safely recommend its use to patients, family members, or friends.

With this book, you'll be able to reassure anxious patients with simple explanations that make sense. And the layman using this guide will find it helpful and easy to understand.

Charlotte Isler, R.N.

Publisher's Notes

Charlotte Isler, R.N., has been a writer and editor with RN Magazine since 1969 and is currently Clinical Editor. She has been both a staff and head nurse in various hospitals and ambulatory-care facilities. In addition to her work with RN Magazine, she has written a number of articles on nursing, medical, and general health-care subjects for various health-care journals, and is the author of *The Nurses' Aide,* published in 1968 by Springer Publishing Company.

How to Use This Dictionary

If you already know the name of the test, simply look it up in the Definitions section, which lists diagnostic tests, procedures, and terms in alphabetical order. There you'll find a brief explanation of each test; the body tissue, fluid, or part examined; and the normal range of values for each result. The units of measure used to express the normal values are explained in the Measures and Equivalents section.

If you know only the abbreviation of a test, procedure, or term, use the alphabetical Abbreviations section in the front of the book as a cross-reference. Each full name listed there with its abbreviation can be looked up in the Definitions section.

The normal values for a given test are not always universally agreed upon. A test result must be interpreted in the context of each individual case. In addition, test results vary depending on the laboratory method and the specific laboratory doing the test. The normal values in this dictionary have been summarized from the best current sources available. They are listed in the Bibliography.

Diagnostic procedures have been included in this book because they are often a necessary prelude to the performance of a laboratory test. Relevant terms have also been included to enhance understanding of the diagnostic tests.

Abbreviations

A

ACG: apexcardiogram

ACTH: adrenocorticotropic hormone

ADNAase: antideoxyribonuclease

AF: amniotic fluid

A/G ratio: albumin/globulin ratio

a-HBD: α-hydroxybutyric dehydrogenase

ALA: aminolevulinic acid

Alb: albumin

Alc: alcohol

Ald: aldolase

Ald assay: aldolase assay

ANA: antinuclear antibodies

Anti-DNAse B: antideoxyribonuclease B

Anti-DS-DNA: anti-doublestranded deoxyribonucleic acid

Anti-ENA: anti-extractable nuclear antigen

APTT: activated partial thromboplastin time

As: arsenic

ASH: antistreptococcal hyaluronidase

ASLO: antistreptolysin O

ATA: antithyroglobulin antibody

AU: Australian antigen

AZ: Aschheim-Zondek test

B

BAO: basal acid output

BCG: Bacillus Calmette-Guerin

BE: barium enema

BE: base excess

Be: beryllium

BEI: butanol-extractable iodine

BG: blood gases

bili: bilirubin

bl cult: blood culture

bleed and CT: bleeding and clotting time

BMR: basal metabolic rate

BSP: Bromsulphalein

BUN: blood urea nitrogen

BX: biopsy

C

C: Celsius

Ca: calcium

Ca: cancer

CA: coccidioidomycosis antibodies

CAT: computerized axial tomography

CBC: complete blood count

CEA: carcinoembryonic antigen

ceph-flocc: cephalin-cholesterol flocculation

CHO: carbohydrate

chol: cholesterol

CI: color index

Cl: chloride

coag: coagulation

CO_2: carbon dioxide

CPK: creatine phosphokinase

CPR: cardiopulmonary resuscitation

creat: creatinine

CRP: C-reactive protein

CSF: cerebrospinal fluid

CT: clotting time

Cu: copper

cult: culture

D

D&C: dilatation and curettage

DHA: dehydroepiandrosterone

diff: differential

DNA: deoxyribonucleic acid

E

EBV: Epstein-Barr virus

ECG: electrocardiogram

EchoEEG: echoencephalogram

EEG: electroencephalogram

EKG: electrocardiogram

EMG: electromyogram

EPI: epinephrine

ER: estrogen receptor

ESR: erythrocyte sedimentation rate

etiol: etiology

F

F: Fahrenheit

Fe: iron

FeBC: iron-binding capacity

FEV: forced expiratory volume, timed

FFA: free fatty acids

FIGLU: formiminoglutamic acid

FSH: follicle-stimulating hormone

FSH & LH: gonadotropins, pituitary (follicle-stimulating hormone and luteinizing hormone)

FTA-ABS: fluorescent treponemal antibody absorption

G

GA: gastric analysis

gal: galactose

GBIA: Guthrie bacterial inhibition assay

GB series: gallbladder series

GF-BAO: gastric fluid, basal acid output

GG: gamma globulin

GGTP: gamma glutamyl transpeptidase

GI series: gastrointestinal series

G-6-PD or G6PD: glucose-6-phosphate dehydrogenase

GTT: glucose tolerance test

H

HAA: hepatitis associated antigen

Hb: hemoglobin

HbA_2: hemoglobin A_2

HBAg: hepatitis B antigen

HbF: hemoglobin F

HCG: human chorionic gonadotropin

HCO_3: carbonate

H_2CO_3: carbonic acid

Hct: hematocrit

Hgb: hemoglobin

HGH: human growth hormone

5-HIAA: 5-hydroxyindoleacetic acid

HL-A: human leukocyte locus A antigen

Hp: haptoglobin

HPL: human placental lactogen

HSV_1: herpes virus type 1

HSV_2: herpes virus type 2

HVA: homovanillic acid

I

IBC: iron-binding capacity

IC: intravascular coagulation

ICDH: isocitric dehydrogenase

IF: intrinsic factor

Ig: immune globulin, immunoglobulin

IM: intramuscular

immunol: immunology

incompat: incompatible

infect: infection

I sat %: iron saturation, percent

isoenz: isoenzyme

IV: intravenous

IVP: intravenous pyelogram

J

jaund: jaundice

K

K: potassium

17-KS: 17-ketosteroids

L

LA: lactic acid

LAP: leucine aminopeptidase

LAP: leukocyte alkaline phosphatase

LATS: long-acting thyroid stimulator

LDH: lactic dehydrogenase

LF: latex fixation

LH: luteinizing hormone

Li: lithium

LP: lumbar puncture

L/S ratio: lecithin/sphingomyelin ratio

LT: lactose tolerance

M

MAO: maximal acid output

MAO: monoamine oxidase

MBC: maximum breathing capacity

MCH: mean corpuscular hemoglobin

MCHC: mean corpuscular hemoglobin concentration

MCV: mean corpuscular volume

metab: metabolism

Mg: magnesium

MIC antibody: microsomal antibody (thyroid)

MIC/MBC: minimal inhibitory concentration/ minimal bactericidal concentration

MMEF: maximum midexpiratory flow

MMPI: Minnesota Multiphasic Personality Inventory

N

N: nitrogen

5′N: 5′-nucleotidase

Na: sodium

NH_3: ammonia

NH_4: ammonium

NPN: nonprotein nitrogen

O

O_2: oxygen

OCT: ornithine carbamoyl transferase

17-OHCS: 17-hydroxycorticosteroids

O&P: ova and parasites

P

P: phosphorus

PAH: para-aminohippuric acid

Pap smear: Papanicolaou smear

Pb: lead

PBI: protein-bound iodine

PC: phenol coefficient

PCG: phonocardiogram

pCO_2: partial pressure of carbon dioxide

PEG: pneumoencephalogram

PgRT: progesterone receptor test

pH: hydrogen ion concentration (acidity or alkalinity)

phos: phosphatase

phy: phytohemagglutinin test

PKU: phenylketonuria

PO_2: partial pressure of oxygen

PO_4: phosphate

PPD: purified protein derivative

PRA: plasma renin activity

PSP: phenolsulfonphthalein

PT: prothrombin time

PTT: partial thromboplastin time

PV: plasma volume

Q

QNS: quantity not sufficient

QRC: quantitative radiocardiography

R

R: roentgen

rad: radiation absorbed dose

RAI: radioactive iodine

RAST: radioimmunosorbent assay test

RBC: red blood cell (count)

rem: roentgen equivalent, man

RF: rheumatoid factor

Rh: Rh factor in blood

RI: refractive index

RIA: radioimmunoassay

RNA: ribonucleic acid

RPG: retrograde pyelogram

RPR: rapid plasma reagin

RT: radiation therapy

RV: residual volume

S

SBT: Simplate bleeding time

SC: subcutaneous

SF: spinal fluid

SF: synovial fluid

SG: specific gravity

SGOT: serum glutamic-oxaloacetic transaminase

SGPT: serum glutamic-pyruvic transaminase

Sig: sigmoidoscopy

SMA: sequential multiple analysis

spec: specimen

sp gr: specific gravity

staph: staphylococcus

strep: streptococcus

stress ECG: stress electrocardiogram

T

T_3: triiodothyronine

T_4: thyroxine

TA: Toxoplasma antibodies

TB: tuberculosis

TBG: thyroxine-binding globulin

TFA: total fatty acids

TG: triglycerides

TGT: thromboplastin generation time

TIBC: total iron-binding capacity

TLC: total lung capacity

TLV: total lung volume

TMA: thyroid microsomal antibody

Tot prot or TP: total proteins

TSH: thyroid-stimulating hormone

TV: total volume

U

UA: uric acid

UCl: urea clearance

Urine spec: urine specimen

US: ultrasound

UU: urinary urobilinogen

UVB_{12}BC: unsaturated vitamin B_{12} binding capacity

V

v: vein

V: venereal

V: ventilation

Vacc: vaccination, vaccine

VC: vital capacity

VCG: vectorcardiogram

VDRL test: Venereal Disease Research Laboratory test

Vect: vector

Vent scan: ventilation scan

Visc: viscous, viscosity

Vit: vitamin

Vit A tol: vitamin A tolerance

VMA: 3-methoxy-4-hydroxymandelic acid (also known as vanillylmandelic acid)

W

WBC: white blood cell (count)

WBC diff: white blood count differential

Wd cult: wound culture

X

X match: crossmatch

XRT: radiation therapy (X-ray therapy)

Z

Zn: zinc

$ZnSO_4$ turb: zinc sulfate turbidity

Measures and Equivalents

Capacity

1 liter (L) =	1,000 milliliters
1 deciliter (dl) =	100 milliliters (1/10 liter)
1 milliliter (ml) =	1/1,000 liter
1 microliter (μl) =	1/1,000,000 liter (1/1,000 milliliter)

Weight

1 kilogram (kg) =	1,000 grams
1 gram (gm) =	1/1,000 kilogram
1 milligram (mg) =	1/1,000 gram
1 microgram (μg, mcg) =	1/1,000,000 gram
1 nanogram (ng) =	1/1,000,000,000 gram
1 picogram (pg) =	1/1,000,000,000,000 gram
1 equivalent (Eq) =	the weight in grams of the amount of an element that replaces or combines with 1 gram of hydrogen
1 milliequivalent (mEq) =	1/1,000 equivalent
1 microequivalent (μEq, microEq) =	1/1,000,000 equivalent

Length

1 meter (m) =	39.37 inches
1 centimeter (cm) =	1/100 meter
1 millimeter (mm) =	1/1,000 meter
1 micrometer (micron, μ) =	1/1,000,000 meter
1 nanometer (nm) =	1/1,000,000,000 meter

Pressure

mm Hg: millimeters of a column of mercury supported by the pressure being measured (used for blood, spinal fluid, and other body fluids)

Concentration

millilgrams percent (mg%): milligrams per 100 cubic centimeters (cc^3) or per 100 grams

volume percent (vol%): the number of milliliters of a substance dissolved in 100 milliliters of a liquid

Mols

mol (M): the weight of a substance in grams, equal to its molecular weight; also called gram molecule, gram molecular weight, and mole

millimol (mM): 1/1,000 mol

milliosmol (mOsm): unit of osmotic pressure exerted by the concentration of an ion in a solution

molar (M) solution: 1 mol of a substance dissolved in 1 liter of solution

Units

unit (U): an arbitrary measurement used in various laboratory techniques and procedures. Cherry-Crandall units, mouse uterine units (MUU), Somogyi units, international units (IU), milli-international units (mIU), Todd units, and the others in this book are unrelated and have different values.

A

Abdominal aortography: X-ray studies of the abdominal aorta and nearby blood vessels after injection of contrast medium directly into the aorta or using various other injection techniques.

Acetaminophen: a drug used to relieve pain and reduce fever. Blood serum levels are measured to monitor therapy, to diagnose overdosage and such toxic reactions as liver damage and coma, and to determine the cause of death in suicide.

Normal values in serum: 5-20 mcg/ml
Two tests are performed: The first is done 4-6 hours after ingestion of the drug; if serum level is high, severe liver damage may result. The second test is done 6-8 hours after ingestion of the drug. If serum level continues to be elevated, hepatic (liver) coma and death may follow.

Acetoacetic acid (in blood): a ketone body produced by metabolic disease or disturbance; also known as diacetic acid.

Normal value in blood: negative

Acetoacetic acid (in urine): a ketone body produced by metabolic disease or disturbance; also known as diacetic acid.

Normal value in urine: negative

Acetone (in blood): a ketone body produced by metabolic disease or disturbance.

Normal value in serum: negative

Acetone (in urine): a ketone body produced by metabolic disease or disturbance.

Normal value in urine: negative

Acidosis: abnormally acid condition of the blood.

Aciduria: abnormally acid urine.

Activated partial thromboplastin time: a blood test to screen for coagulation (blood clotting) disorders, and to determine the adequacy of various clotting factors.

Normal values in venous blood: 32-51 seconds

Addis count: a test done on urine to detect kidney disease.

Normal values in urine after 12-hour collection:
WBC and epithelial cells—1,800,000; RBC—500,000;
Hyaline casts—0-5,000

Adrenaline: *see* Epinephrine.

Adrenocorticotropic hormone: a pituitary hormone that stimulates the adrenal cortex.

Aerobic organism (aerobe): a microorganism that requires atmospheric oxygen in order to grow.

Agar: a substance used in the laboratory to culture microorganisms.

Agglutination: a process in which cells suspended in fluid clump together and become visible to the naked eye.

Agglutinins: antibodies that produce agglutination (clumping) of various types of cells.

Agglutinogen: an antigen that stimulates the production of agglutinins.

Albumin (in blood): a protein elevated in blood in the presence of kidney or various other diseases.

Normal values in serum: 3.2-5.6 gm/dl

Albumin (in cerebrospinal fluid): a protein elevated in CSF in the presence of infection or other disease.

Normal values in CSF: 10-30 mg/dl

Albumin (in urine): a protein in urine found in appreciable amounts only in the presence of kidney or various other diseases.

Normal values in urine: negative to trace, qualitative; after 24-hour collection—negative, or 10-100 mg, quantitative

Albumin/globulin ratio (in blood): the ratio of albumin to globulin; lowered in certain pathological conditions.

Normal values in plasma or serum: 1.3/1 to 3.0/1

Albumin/globulin ratio (in cerebrospinal fluid): the ratio of albumin to globulin; altered in certain disease states such as multiple myeloma.

Normal value in CSF: 1.6/2.2

Alcohol: an intoxicating agent present in blood after ingestion.

Normal value in serum or whole blood: negative

Aldolase assay: a test to determine blood levels of aldolase, an enzyme that converts sugar to energy in the muscles. It is elevated in various conditions including liver necrosis, skeletal muscle disease, granulocytic leukemia, and muscular dystrophy.

Normal values in serum: 0-12 units/ml
(varies by laboratory method)

Aldosterone: a steroid hormone important to electrolyte balance.

Normal values in urine after 24-hour collection: 5-19 mcg

Aliquot: a small, measured sample of body or other fluid.

Alkaptone bodies: a class of substances, especially homogentisic acid, present in urine in alkaptonuria, a rare metabolic disease.

Normal value in urine: negative

Allergen: a substance capable of causing allergy in a susceptible person.

Allergy: hypersensitivity to a specific substance.

Ameba (amoeba): a one-celled protozoan organism that moves via projections called pseudopods.

Amino acid: component of body protein.

α-**Amino acid nitrogen:** a substance measured in urine to diagnose various metabolic disturbances.

Normal values in urine after 24-hour collection: 50-200 mg

Aminoaciduria: excessive amounts of one or more amino acids in the urine.

α-Amino-*n*-butyric acid: a substance present in the blood of heavy drinkers of alcohol.

Normal value in blood: negative

Aminoglycoside serum assay: a blood test done to make sure that antibiotic drugs such as gentamicin (Garamycin), tobramycin (Nebcin), and amikacin (Amikin) are administered in dosages that maintain therapeutic blood levels.

Normal values (for therapeutic levels in whole blood drawn 30 minutes after IV or 60 minutes after IM administration—peak level, and just before next dose—trough level): gentamicin and tobramycin—4-10 mcg/ml; amikacin—15-35 mcg/ml

δ-Aminolevulinic acid (in blood): a protein product of metabolism, measured in blood to diagnose lead poisoning or porphyria, a blood disease.

Normal values in serum: 0.01-0.03 mg/dl

δ-Aminolevulinic acid (in urine): a protein product of metabolism, measured in urine to diagnose lead poisoning.

Normal values in urine (random): adults—0.1-0.6 mg/dl; children—less than 0.5 mg/dl

Normal values in urine after 24-hour collection: 1.5-7.5 mg

Ammonia: a substance produced by bacterial activity in the intestine; measured in blood to determine adequate liver function in converting ammonia into

Continued

urea, a substance excreted by the kidneys. Serum ammonia levels rise in liver disease and are useful in diagnosing impending or already established hepatic coma, as well as for monitoring treatment. Elevated serum ammonia levels may also be helpful in diagnosing Reye's syndrome.

Normal values in venous or arterial blood:
40-70 mcg/100 ml

Normal values in plasma: 20-150 mcg/dl
(by diffusion method)

Ammonia nitrogen: a substance measured in urine to determine the body's acid/base balance and nitrogen balance.

Normal values in urine (random): 35-70 mcg/dl

Normal values in urine after 24-hour collection:
20-70 mEq; 500-1200 mg

Amniocentesis: insertion of a needle through the abdomen into a pregnant woman's uterus to obtain a sample of amniotic fluid (the fluid that surrounds the fetus) for detection of the sex and various genetic factors or diseases of the unborn child.

Amniotic fluid, absorbance difference at 450 nm: a test done on amniotic fluid via spectrophotometry to detect fetal blood abnormalities in early or late pregnancy.

Normal values in AF: early pregnancy—less than 0.05 optical density difference (O.D.D.); at term—less than 0.02 O.D.D.

Amniotic fluid, appearance: a test for normal visual appearance of the amniotic fluid in early or late pregnancy.

Normal values in AF: early pregnancy, before 28 weeks—clear; at term—clear or slightly opalescent

Amniotic fluid, bilirubin: a test done on amniotic fluid to detect fetal abnormalities, such as hemolytic disease, in early or late pregnancy.

Normal values in AF: early pregnancy—less than 0.075 mg/dl; at term—less than 0.025 mg/dl

Amniotic fluid, chloride: an amniotic fluid test to detect fetal problems in early or late pregnancy.

Normal values in AF: early pregnancy—about equal to serum chloride; at term—generally lower than serum chloride

Amniotic fluid, creatinine: a test done on amniotic fluid to determine the age of the fetus.

Normal values in AF: early pregnancy—0.8-1.1 mg/dl; at term—1.8-4.0 mg/dl, usually more than 2.0 mg/dl

Amniotic fluid, cytologic staining (Nile blue sulfate): a count of fat-staining cells in a sample of amniotic fluid; done to determine the age of the fetus.

Normal values in AF: early pregnancy—less than 2% of total cells; at term—20% or more of total cells

Amniotic fluid, estriol: a test done on amniotic fluid to detect fetal abnormalities, such as fetoplacental depression, in early or late pregnancy.

Normal values in AF: early pregnancy—less than 10 mcg/dl; at term—more than 60 mcg/dl

Amniotic fluid, lecithin/sphingomyelin ratio: the ratio of two components of AF, found to be a predictor of fetal lung maturity.

Normal value in AF: 2/1 or greater

Amniotic fluid, osmolality: a test done on amniotic fluid to detect fetal abnormalities in early or late pregnancy.

Normal values in AF: early pregnancy—about equal to serum osmolality; at term—less than 250 mOsm/liter

Amniotic fluid, pCO_2: measurement of the partial pressure of carbon dioxide in amniotic fluid; done to detect fetal abnormalities in early or late pregnancy.

Normal values in AF: early pregnancy—33-55 mm Hg; at term—42-55 mm Hg (increases toward term)

Amniotic fluid, pH: measurement of acidity or alkalinity of amniotic fluid; done to detect fetal distress, or other fetal abnormalities, in early or late pregnancy.

Normal values in AF: early pregnancy—7.12-7.38; at term—6.91-7.43 (decreases toward term)

Amniotic fluid, rapid surfactant test: *see* Rapid surfactant test.

Amniotic fluid, sodium: an amniotic fluid test to detect fetal problems in early or late pregnancy.

Normal values in AF: early pregnancy—about equal to serum sodium; at term—about 7-10 mEq/liter lower than serum sodium

Amniotic fluid, total protein: a test done on amniotic fluid to detect fetal abnormalities in early or late pregnancy.

Normal values in AF: early pregnancy—0.60 ± 0.24 gm/dl; at term—0.26 ± 0.19 gm/dl

Amniotic fluid, urea: a test done on amniotic fluid to detect fetal problems in early or late pregnancy.

Normal values in AF: early pregnancy—18.0 ± 5.9 mg/dl; at term—30.3 ± 11.4 mg/dl

Amniotic fluid, uric acid: an amniotic fluid test to detect fetal problems in early or late pregnancy.

Normal values in AF: early pregnancy—3.72 ± 0.96 mg/dl; at term—9.9 ± 2.23 mg/dl

Amniotic fluid, volume: measurement of amniotic fluid volume to detect fetal abnormalities in early or late pregnancy.

Normal values in AF: early pregnancy—450-1200 ml; at term—500-1400 ml (increases toward term)

Amylase (in blood): an enzyme secreted by the pancreas; elevated in disease of the pancreas or salivary glands, kidney problems, and drug ingestion.

Normal values in serum: 60-150 Somogyi units/100 ml

Amylase (in urine): an enzyme secreted by the pancreas; elevated in urine in the presence of pancreatitis due to mumps or other cause.

Normal values in urine after 24-hour collection:
1,000-5,000 Somogyi units

Anaerobic organism (anaerobe): a microorganism that can grow only in the absence of atmospheric oxygen.

Anaphylaxis: an extreme allergic state that may be fatal if not treated immediately.

Androsterone: a sex hormone secreted by the testes and the adrenal glands.

Normal values in urine after 24-hour collection:
males—2.8-5.0 mg; females—0.8-3.0 mg

Angiocardiogram: a radiographic record of the internal structure of the heart and great blood vessels (pulmonary arteries, veins, and the aorta) after injection of contrast medium.

Angiogram: a radiographic record of the internal structure of blood vessels after injection of contrast medium.

Angiography: X-ray examination of the blood vessels after injection of contrast medium.

Antibacterial serum: serum that can kill bacteria or prevent their growth.

Antibiotic, serum killing level test: an immunologic test that determines the drug level in serum at which an antibiotic drug can inhibit the growth of or kill a given infectious microorganism.

Adequate values: serum can be diluted 1:8 or more and is still capable of killing the microorganism causing the infection.

Antibody: a protein substance in blood that can kill, or render harmless, invading material (such as disease-causing microorganisms) that might cause infection or other damage.

Anticoagulant: a substance that prevents or delays clotting of blood cells.

Antideoxyribonuclease: an antibody substance measured in blood to detect streptococcal infection.

Normal values in serum: titer of less than 1:20

Antideoxyribonuclease B: an antibody that is measured in blood to diagnose diseases such as rheumatic fever or poststreptococcal glomerulonephritis (kidney disease).

Normal values in whole blood: small children—120 units; older children and adults—1,360 units

Anti-doublestranded deoxyribonucleic acid: an antibody substance measured in blood to help diagnose the presence, and monitor the progress, of systemic lupus erythematosus.

Normal value in whole blood: 15 units/ml

Anti-extractable nuclear antigen: an antibody substance measured in blood to aid in the diagnosis of rheumatic diseases.

Normal value in whole blood: negative

Antigen: a substance in blood capable of inducing the production of antibodies.

Antinuclear antibodies: antibody substances measured in blood to detect a wide variety of diseases, including connective tissue disease; drug-associated disease; and others involving the liver, intestines, and circulatory system.

Normal values in serum: titer of less than 1:10

Antiseptic: a substance that checks, or prevents, the growth of microorganisms.

Antiserum: serum that has immune properties (contains antibodies).

Antistreptococcal hyaluronidase: an antibody substance measured in blood to detect streptococcal infection.

Normal values in serum: titer of less than 1:256

Antistreptolysin O: an antibody substance measured in blood to detect streptococcal infection.

Normal values in serum: less than 160 Todd units

Antithyroglobulin antibody: a thyroid autoantibody, present in patients with autoimmune reactions in the thyroid gland.

Normal values in serum: titer of less than 1:32

Antitoxin: immune serum that neutralizes or prevents harmful action by a toxin (a poisonous substance produced by disease-causing microorganisms).

Aortoarteriography: X-ray studies, using a series of films, of the circulatory system of the abdomen and a portion of the lower extremities, after injecting contrast medium through a needle or catheter into an artery or vein in the lower part of the body.

Apexcardiography: a procedure in which a transducer is applied to the apex of the heart (the lowest point of the heart that is also the farthest to the left), to identify abnormal heart sounds in such conditions as heart valve disease or tumor of the heart muscle.

Argininosuccinic lyase: an enzyme used to measure liver function.

Normal values in serum: 0-4 U/dl

Arsenic (in blood): a toxic substance found in the blood in arsenic poisoning.

Normal values in blood: less than 3 mcg/dl

Arsenic (in urine): a toxic substance found in the urine in arsenic poisoning.

Normal values in urine after 24-hour collection:
less than 50 mcg/liter

Arteriography: X-ray studies of the structure of one or more arteries and other nearby blood vessels after injection of contrast medium.

Arthrography: X-ray studies of one or more joints, using contrast medium to outline the space within the joint.

Arthroscopy: Direct examination of the interior of a joint by means of an arthroscope.

Aschheim-Zondek test: a test for pregnancy (now largely superseded by other tests).

Ascorbic acid (in blood): vitamin C—essential for proper body functioning; deficiency causes scurvy.

Normal values: in plasma—0.6-2.0 mg/dl;
in whole blood—0.7-2.0 mg/dl

Ascorbic acid (in urine): vitamin C—essential for proper body functioning; deficiency causes scurvy.

Normal values in urine: random—1-7 mg/dl; after 24-hour collection—more than 50 mg

Ascorbic acid tolerance: a test to determine the extent of ascorbic acid deficiency; blood levels are measured following administration of a known amount of vitamin C.

Normal values in plasma: 1.6 mg/dl or more

Aseptic: sterile.

Aspirate: fluid drawn by suction from the body for lab examination, or to reduce excess fluid.

Atomic absorption spectrophotometry: a technique for measuring trace elements (for example, calcium, magnesium, copper) in body fluids.

Atrophy: a reduction in size of a body part due to illness or other wasting condition.

Audiometry: a test to measure hearing functions.

Australian antigen: an antigen often found in the serum of people who have had hepatitis; the blood test for this antigen is used to detect serum hepatitis (type B), and to differentiate it from type A hepatitis.

Normal value in serum: negative, but sometimes present in otherwise healthy Americans and in many people who live in the Middle East and Asia.

Autoantibody: an antibody that acts like a foreign substance and may react against normal tissues to cause disease.

Autoantigen: a self-produced antigen that induces antibody production.

Autoclave: a machine that sterilizes objects and equipment using pressurized steam.

Autogenous vaccine: a vaccine produced by culturing a patient's own bacteria.

Autoimmune disease: disease in which the body produces an immune response against itself.

Autoimmunity: a condition that occurs when a patient's antibodies attack his own body proteins.

Autoinfection: infection transferred from an infected body part to one or more additional parts.

Autolysis: destruction of cells by body enzymes.

Autopsy: the external and internal examination of the body after death.

Avitaminosis: a deficiency state due to severe lack of essential vitamins.

Azygography: radiographic examination of the azygos vein system (posterior chest) after injection of contrast medium.

B

Bacillus Calmette-Guerin: a bovine tubercle microorganism used in a vaccine that protects against tuberculosis.

Bacteremia: contamination of the bloodstream with bacteria.

Bacterial sensitivity test: a laboratory procedure to determine which antibiotic drug will most effectively counteract a specific infection.

Bactericide: an agent that kills bacteria.

Bacteriology: the science of bacteria.

Bacteriolysins: antibodies that dissolve bacteria when complement (a normal body protein needed for antigen/antibody reaction) is present.

Bacteriophage: a virus that causes disintegration of bacteria.

Bacteriostasis: a condition that inhibits the growth of bacteria without necessarily killing them.

Barbiturates: a class of sedative drugs; barbiturate blood levels are measured in patients who have taken overdoses either accidentally, to abuse drugs, or to commit suicide.

Normal value in serum, plasma, or whole blood: negative

Barium enema: the use of barium sulfate and air as contrast media to help with visualization of the interior of the colon in X-ray studies.

Basal acid output: *see under* Gastric fluid.

Basal metabolic rate: a measurement of thyroid function, via a breathing test that measures oxygen used and calories spent while the body is at rest.

Normal values: from 15% less to 15% more than a person of the same age, sex, height, and weight would use at rest.

Base excess: a test of the body's acid-base balance, measured as bicarbonate.

Normal values in serum: 24-26 mEq/liter

Bedside radiography: X-ray studies performed at the bedside when the patient is too ill to be moved.

Bence Jones protein: a protein excreted in urine in the presence of various conditions, such as multiple myeloma.

Normal value in urine: negative

Benign condition: an abnormal condition that is not malignant.

Beryllium: an element not normally present in urine except in very small quantities.

Normal values in urine after 24-hour collection: less than 0.05 mcg

Bicarbonate: a constituent of carbonic acid; blood levels of bicarbonate provide an index of the body's alkali reserve.

Normal values in plasma: 24-26 mEq/liter

Bilirubin (in blood): a substance formed during the breakdown of hemoglobin; measured in the blood in liver disease, gallbladder disease, and various types of anemia.

Normal values in plasma or serum: total—0.2-1.5 mg/dl; direct—0.1-0.4 mg/dl; indirect—0.1-1.0 mg/dl; newborns, total—1.0-12 mg/dl

Bilirubin (in urine): a substance formed during the breakdown of hemoglobin in the blood; present in urine in conditions such as obstructive disease of the gallbladder or liver disease.

Normal value in urine: negative

Biopsy: the surgical removal of body tissue for microscopic examination.

Biplane cerebral angiography: X-ray studies of the blood vessels in the brain after injection of contrast medium, showing the structures from the side (laterally) and front-to-back (anteroposteriorly).

Bleeding and clotting time: two blood tests, generally performed at the same time, to show how rapidly the small blood vessels constrict to stop bleeding, and how effectively the blood's clotting mechanisms are working.

Normal values: bleeding—3-10 minutes (depending on method used); clotting—5-15 minutes

Blood culture: the incubation of a blood sample in nutrient material to determine the growth and type of infection-causing microorganisms.

Normal value in blood: negative for microorganisms

Blood gases: gases dissolved in the blood that maintain its acid-base balance. *See also* Partial pressure; pH.

Blood, occult (in feces): small amounts of blood found in the feces when an abnormality is present somewhere in the intestinal tract; used to detect injury or diseases such as cancer, anemia, and infection.

Normal value in feces: negative

Blood, occult (in urine): small amounts of blood found in the urine in disease of the kidney or urinary tract, or following trauma.

Normal value in urine: negative

Blood-synovial fluid glucose difference: *see under* Synovial fluid.

Blood type: the type and subtype of an individual's blood; specified as A, B, AB, or O; Rh-negative or Rh-positive; and including a number of subtypes. It is important to determine the blood type when a woman is pregnant, or when a patient needs a transfusion, in order to avoid a dangerous reaction with an incompatible type.

Blood urea nitrogen: *see* Urea nitrogen.

Blood volume: a measure of a patient's total blood volume.

Normal values for whole blood: males—69 ml/kg; females—65 ml/kg

---

B lymphocytes: lymphocytes (lymph cells) that are bone-marrow-dependent (originate in the bone marrow), and function as part of the immune system to protect against infection.

Bone marrow aspiration: removal of bone marrow from the breastbone or hipbone by aspiration through a needle. The blood cells produced by the bone marrow are evaluated as to number, appearance, development, and presence of infection. Done when leukemia, anemia, or other disease affecting the bone marrow is suspected.

Normal values in bone marrow: some 15 different types of cells in given numbers and stages of maturation, as evaluated by a hematologist (blood specialist).

Bone scan: a scan of the bones after injection of radioactive material into a vein. An increased concentration of radioactive material in a given area may indicate cancer, arthritis, fracture, or other disease conditions.

Bone X-ray: X-ray studies of bone to determine if fracture or disease is present.

Brain scan: a scan of the brain after injection of radioactive material into a vein. An increased concentration of radioactive material in a given area indicates pathology. The test is done twice: immediately after the injection, and again 24 hours later.

Broad-spectrum antibiotic: one that is effective against a wide range of microorganisms.

Bromides: a chemical class found in over-the-counter sedative medications and in some prescription drugs. Blood levels are measured to detect toxicity.

Normal values in serum: negative; therapeutic levels—0-5 mg/dl

Bromsulphalein: a chemical used in liver function tests. It is injected intravenously and its retention in the blood is measured after a period of time.

Normal values in serum: less than 6% retention after 45 minutes

Bronchogram: radiographic record of the bronchi and bronchioles after injection of contrast medium.

Bronchoscopy: examination of the bronchi by direct visualization through a bronchoscope, to diagnose abnormalities. The scope may be inserted through the mouth, or directly into the trachea via a tracheostomy (surgical opening in the trachea).

Brucella agglutinins: antibodies elevated in blood of patients with brucellosis.

Normal values in serum: titer of less than 1:80

Buccal smear: cells scraped from the inside of the cheek to detect abnormalities of sexual development.

Continued

Normal values: males—46 chromosomes including one X and one Y, no Barr body; females—46 chromosomes including two X chromosomes, one of which appears as a Barr body

Buffer: a substance that reduces, or prevents, excess acid or alkali in the body.

Calcium: (in blood): a mineral essential for a number of biochemical functions, including transmission of nerve impulses and muscle contractions.

Normal values in serum: 8.5-10.5 mg/dl

Calcium (in cerebrospinal fluid): a mineral with abnormal levels in CSF in the presence of infections such as tuberculous meningitis.

Normal values in CSF: 2.1-2.9 mEq/liter

Calcium, qualitative: an estimate of the level of calcium in urine, decreased in glandular and nutritional deficiency, increased in patients taking certain diuretic drugs and in some other conditions.

Normal value in urine: 1+ turbidity

Calcium, quantitative: measurement of calcium levels in the urine, decreased in glandular or nutritional deficiency.

Normal values in urine after 24-hour collection: average diet—100-250 mg; low-calcium diet—less than 150 mg; high-calcium diet—250-300 mg

---

Caloric test: a test of the inner ear in which hot water or ice water is instilled in the ear and eye movement observed; performed on patients with ear disease or injury, or symptoms of dizziness or fainting.

Continued

Caloric test

Normal values: eye movement toward the site of hot water instillation; away from the site of ice water instillation

---

Capillary fragility test: a test to measure the fragility of small blood vessels near the skin; done with a blood pressure cuff. Fragility of these vessels is indicative of various blood vessel diseases.

Carbohydrates: a class of organic compounds of carbon combined with hydrogen and oxygen, the latter two in the same proportion as in water. The class includes sugars, starches, and cellulose.

Carbon dioxide combining power: a blood test that measures the carbon dioxide absorbed at a given pressure and temperature; done in respiratory and other problems.

Normal values in venous plasma or serum:
24-30 mM/liter; 50-58 vol%

Carbon dioxide content: measurement of carbonic acid and bicarbonate in blood, plasma, or serum; done in respiratory problems.

Normal values: in whole blood—19-24 mM/liter;
in arterial plasma or serum—21-28 mM/liter;
in venous whole blood—22-26 mM/liter;
in venous plasma or serum—24-30 mM/liter

Carbonic acid: an acid that results from dissolving carbon dioxide in water; blood levels are measured to determine respiratory function.

Normal values: in arterial whole blood—1.05-1.45 mM/liter; in venous whole blood—1.15-1.50 mM/liter; in venous plasma—1.02-1.38 mM/liter

---

Carboxyhemoglobin: a compound of carbon monoxide and hemoglobin. Carbon monoxide poisoning is detected by measuring the capacity of the heme portion of the hemoglobin (Hgb) molecule to combine with carbon monoxide.

Normal values in whole blood: in suburban non-smokers—less than 1.5% saturation of Hgb; in smokers—1.5-5.0%; in heavy smokers—5.0-9.0%

Carcinoembryonic antigen: an antigen measured in serum and sometimes other body fluids to detect the presence or recurrence of cancer in such sites as the colon, pancreas, lung, breast, or prostate.

Normal values in serum: less than 2 ng/ml; and in very small quantities in pregnant women, normal adults, and infants

---

Cardiac catheterization: *see under* Heart.

Cardiopulmonary resuscitation: the restoration of heartbeat and breathing by external cardiac compression and mouth-to-mouth breathing.

Carotene: a precursor of vitamin A; blood levels are measured in patients with night blindness and other forms of vitamin A deficiency.

Normal values in serum: 40-200 mcg/dl

Carotid arteriography: X-ray studies of the neck arteries after injection of contrast medium into the carotid artery.

Carrier: an otherwise healthy person who harbors disease-causing organisms that may be transmitted to others.

Catabolism: the process of breakdown of complex body compounds into simpler ones.

Catalyst: a substance that promotes or speeds up a chemical reaction, but is not changed in the process.

Catecholamines: compounds, such as adrenaline and noradrenaline, produced by the medulla (central portion) of the adrenal glands. Catecholamines may be elevated after ingestion of coffee, bananas, and certain drugs, and in patients with pheochromocytoma, a tumor of the adrenal gland.

Normal values in urine: random—0-14 mcg/dl; after 24-hour collection—less than 100 mcg (can vary with activity)

Catheterization, cardiac: *see under* Heart.

Catheterization, urinary: a procedure in which a sterile thin tube (catheter) is passed into the urinary bladder, either to remove urine when the patient cannot urinate normally or to obtain sterile urine for diagnostic tests.

Catheterized urine specimen: a urine specimen obtained through a catheter under sterile conditions, protected from contamination by organisms elsewhere in or on the patient's body, or on the hands of the person obtaining the specimen. Such a specimen can be tested for microorganisms in the urinary tract.

Celiac angiography: X-ray studies of the blood vessels of the liver, spleen, stomach, and pancreas after injection of contrast medium.

Cell culture: the process of growing cells in a nutrient solution or material outside the body.

Cellulitis: inflammation of connective tissues.

Celsius (centigrade): a temperature scale on which 0° is the freezing point of water, and 100° is the boiling point of water.

Cephalin-cholesterol flocculation test: a test for liver disease, based on reaction in mixture of patient's serum with an emulsion of cephalin and cholesterol.

Normal values in serum: negative to 1+ after 24 hours; 2+ or less after 48 hours.

Cerebral angiography: X-ray studies of cerebral blood vessels after injection of contrast medium.

Cerebrospinal fluid: the fluid that bathes the brain and spinal canal. It may be examined for the presence of blood, infection, and other abnormalities.

Normal values: listed under CSF constituents

Cerebrospinal fluid, cell count: a test to detect infection in the brain or spinal canal.

Normal values in CSF: 0-8 cells/microliter

Cerebrospinal fluid culture: incubation of a sample of CSF in the laboratory to determine whether it contains disease-causing microorganisms.

Cerebrospinal fluid scan: scan of the brain after injection of a radioactive substance into the spinal canal; done to detect spinal fluid leak or abnormalities of the skull.

Ceruloplasmin: a protein with which most of the blood's copper is combined. Elevated levels may occur in liver disease, leukemia, and heart attack. Decreased levels occur in other forms of liver disease, and in nutritional deficiencies.

Normal values in serum: 23-50 mg/dl

Cerumen: earwax.

Chest X-ray: an X-ray to detect lung disease, or determine the size and position of the heart, ribs, or other internal structures of the chest.

Chloride (in blood): a salt that provides diagnostic information on the blood's acid-base balance, osmotic status, and water balance.

Normal values in serum: 95-103 mEq/liter

Chloride (in cerebrospinal fluid): a salt that is measured in CSF to detect brain or spinal infection or other abnormalities.

Normal values in CSF: adult—118-132 mEq/liter; children—120-128 mEq/liter

---

Chloride (in sweat): a salt elevated in sweat in patients with fibrocystic disease.

Normal values in sweat: 4-60 mEq/liter

Chloride (in urine): a salt elevated in urine in drug toxicity, dehydration, and some forms of kidney disease; decreased with excessive excretion of urine, sweating, diarrhea, or vomiting.

Normal values in urine after 24-hour collection:
110-250 mEq/liter

Cholangiography: X-ray studies of the gallbladder and ducts often done in the course of surgery of the gallbladder and related structures.

Cholecystography, oral: radiographic examination of the gallbladder, done after the patient eats a prepared fatty meal, and swallows a contrast agent (usually pills) that outlines the gallbladder and nearby structures.

Cholesterol: a steroid found in animal tissues and body fluids, important in various metabolic processes, and implicated as a factor in arteriosclerosis.

Cholesterol, total: a measurement of the blood levels of cholesterol, elevated in certain liver, thyroid, kidney, and other diseases; decreased in certain anemias, glandular deficiencies, and other forms of liver disease.

Normal values in serum: 150-250 mg/dl, depending on diet and age

---

Cholinesterase: a catalytic enzyme that hydrolyzes acetylcholine into choline and acetic acid; it is needed for transmission of nerve impulses of the parasympathetic nervous system. Decreased levels may indicate organic phosphate poisoning, cancer, liver and certain skin conditions.

Normal values in erythrocytes (red blood cells):
0.65-1.00 pH units/ml

Chromatin: the part of a cell's nucleus that can be stained.

Chromatography: a chemical analysis technique in which substances such as hormones, drugs, or enzymes are first separated and then identified by passing them through an adsorbent.

Chromogenic: capable of producing color.

Chromosome: a threadlike body in the nucleus of a living cell that transmits hereditary characteristics.

Chromosome analysis: a test done on white blood cells, bone marrow, or skin cells that have been prepared and chemically treated, for detection of sex identity and various genetic diseases, such as mongolism (Down's syndrome), in the fetus, child, or adult.

Cineradiography: a process in which fluoroscopic images of moving body parts are projected on an image intensifier, then photographed for viewing as a videotape on a television screen.

Citrate agar hemoglobin electrophoresis: a procedure that separates and identifies various forms of hemoglobin, such as HbA or HbF. HbF is the primary hemoglobin type found in newborns. A high HbF concentration in adults may indicate early hereditary anemia. Presence of HbS indicates sickle-cell anemia.

Normal values in venous blood (adults): HbA_1—97-98% of total hemoglobin; HbA_2—1.5-3.5%; HbF—less than 2%; HbS—none

Citric acid: a compound similar to ascorbic acid (vitamin C).

Normal values in serum or plasma: 1.7-3.0 mg/dl

Clone: the reproduction of a cell in its exact image.

Clotting time: *see* Bleeding and clotting time.

Coagulase: an enzyme that speeds the clotting process in blood.

Coagulation: the process of clotting, or clumping of blood.

Coagulation tests: tests performed on whole blood, plasma, or serum to determine the blood's capacity to clot. Abnormal results indicate coagulation defects due to disease or medication.

Normal values in blood:
bleeding time: 3-10 minutes (depending on method used)
clot retraction: half of the original mass in 2 hours
dilute blood clot lysis time: 6-10 hours at 37° C
euglobulin lysis time: 2-6 hours at 37° C
venous clotting time, 3 tubes: 5-15 minutes
whole blood clot lysis time: none in 24 hours
prothrombin time: 12-14 seconds
partial thromboplastin time: 60-85 seconds (after addition of partial thromboplastin reagent and ionized calcium)

Coccidioidomycosis antibodies: antibodies that are found in the blood of patients with coccidioidomycosis, a fungus infection that affects the respiratory tract and occasionally other parts of the body such as skin, bone, and central nervous system.

Normal value in serum: negative

Coccus: a type of bacterial cell.

Cofactor: a substance that is essential to the function of an enzyme.

Cold agglutinins: agglutinins that act only at low temperatures; present in the blood of patients with atypical pneumonia. Using the agglutination process, a distinction may be made between Mycoplasma and virus pneumonia.

Normal values in serum: titer of less than 1:32

Coliform bacteria: bacteria, such as Escherichia coli, that live in the intestine.

Colonoscopy: examination of the colon by inserting a flexible instrument called a fiberoptic endoscope. The endoscope is used to visualize abnormalities along the entire length of the colon and to remove diagnostic tissue samples and small growths.

Colony: a large group of microorganisms grown in a culture medium from a small sample; used for diagnostic purposes or for making vaccines and other preparations for treatment or prevention of disease.

Combined fatty acids test: a test done on feces to determine the patient's ability to digest fats.

Normal values in feces: 5%-15% of dry matter

Communicable disease: a disease that can be transmitted from one person to another through direct contact, air vectors, food, body fluids, or excreta.

Complement: a blood protein capable of killing bacteria and other cells or organisms in the presence of an antigen-antibody complex.

Complement C3: a complement component with elevated blood levels in cancer, and decreased blood levels in kidney disease, liver disease, and severe allergic reactions.

Normal values in serum: 100-170 mg/dl

Complement fixation: the binding of complement by an antigen-antibody complex. This reaction is the basis of diagnostic tests for virus infection, fungus-caused lung disease, and a number of other infectious diseases.

Complete blood count: a blood test to determine the number of red and white blood cells, and the concentration (hematocrit) and quality of the red cells in a sample of blood.

Normal values in whole blood:
hematocrit: males, 40-54%; females, 38-47%
hemoglobin: males, 13.5-18 gm/dl; females, 12.0-16 gm/dl
red cell count: males, 4.6-6.2 million/mm^3; females, 4.2-5.4 million/mm^3
white cell count: 4,500-11,000/mm^3

Compound F: *see* Cortisol.

Computerized axial tomography: a radiologic technique in which a radioactive isotope is injected, and the radioactive emissions are picked up by the scanning apparatus and transmitted to a computer. An image of the scanned body part is then reconstructed on the screen of a video display terminal.

Concentration test: a test of the kidney's capacity to concentrate and dilute urine.

Normal values in random urine specimen after fluid restriction: specific gravity—more than 1.025; osmolality—more than 850 mOsm/liter

---

Conization: removal of conical piece of tissue.

Contrast medium: a liquid or semisolid substance that is radiopaque (won't allow the passage of X-rays through it); used to make internal structures visible during radiologic examinations and on X-ray film.

Convalescent carrier: a person or animal recovering from an infection but still harboring the disease-causing microorganisms, and capable of transmitting them to others.

Convalescent serum: the serum of a person who has recovered from an infection. It may be given to another person as a preventive measure.

Coombs's test: a test to detect, and differentiate between, various types of anemias; most commonly used to detect blood incompatibility reactions in pregnant women and their babies.

Normal values: direct (in cord blood)—no antibodies coating the red blood cells (no complete agglutination); indirect (in maternal serum)—no antibodies to red blood cell antigens.

Copper (in blood): a mineral essential for hemoglobin synthesis.

Normal values in serum or plasma: male—70-140 mcg/dl; female—85-155 mcg/dl

Copper (in urine): a mineral excreted in urine in increased amounts in certain liver diseases, infections, heart attacks, and leukemia, and in decreased amounts in Wilson's disease and sprue.

Normal values in urine after 24-hour collection: 0-30 mcg

Coproantibodies: antibodies produced in the intestinal tract.

Coproporphyrin: a substance normally excreted in urine in minute amounts, and elevated in liver and certain metabolic diseases.

Normal values in urine (random): adults—3-20 mcg/10 ml

Normal values in urine after 24-hour collection: adults—50-250 mcg; children—0-80 mcg

---

Coprozoic: found in feces.

Coronary arteriography: X-ray studies of the coronary arteries after injection of contrast medium through a catheter.

Cortisol (compound F, hydrocortisone): a principal secretion of the cortex (outer layer) of the adrenal glands; blood levels are measured to detect Addison's disease, adrenogenital syndrome, Cushing's syndrome, and other conditions.

Normal values in plasma: in AM—5-25 mcg/dl;
in PM—2-18 mcg/dl

Counterstain: a second stain applied over a first for greater staining effect.

C-peptide test: a test done on diabetic patients to determine if they are able to make their own insulin.

Normal value in blood: C-peptide is present

C-reactive protein: a protein found in the blood of patients with inflammatory diseases; its presence can help determine the cause of rheumatoid arthritis and certain types of pneumonias or other upper respiratory infections.

Normal value in serum: negative

Creatine: a compound normally stored in muscle tissue as phosphocreatine and found in small quantities in urine.

Normal values in urine after 24-hour collection: males—0-40 mg; females—0-100 mg; higher in children and during pregnancy

Creatine phosphokinase: an enzyme present in the heart and skeletal muscles. Blood levels are elevated following a heart attack and in patients with muscular dystrophy and other muscle conditions.

Normal values in serum: males—55-170 U/liter at 37°C; females—30-135 U/liter at 37°C

Creatinine: a protein waste product; elevated in disturbances of kidney function.

Normal values in urine after 24-hour collection: males—20-26 mg/kg of body weight; females—14-22 mg/kg of body weight

Creatinine clearance, endogenous: rate at which kidney removes creatinine from the blood; tested to evaluate kidney function.

Normal values in urine: 115 ± 20 ml/minute

Crossmatching: determining compatibility of donor's blood with recipient's blood prior to blood transfusion.

Continued

Normal values in blood: no sign of agglutination (clumping) or hemolysis (destruction) of red blood cells

Cryobiology: the science of biologic effects of very low temperatures.

Cryoglobulins: immunoglobulins that precipitate only in cold temperatures; found mainly in the presence of blood vessel illness.

Normal value in serum: negative

Culture: the incubation of a sample of body fluid in a nutrient broth in order to identify microorganisms.

Culture medium: the nourishing substance used to grow microorganisms in the laboratory.

Cysteine and cystine: amino acids (protein components); elevated in certain metabolic disturbances that can produce kidney and other diseases.

Normal values in urine after 24-hour collection: 10-100 mg

Cystine (quantitative): a urine test for cystine, rarely found except in patients with certain forms of congenital disease.

Normal value in urine: negative

Cystoscopy: direct visual examination of the bladder and part of the urinary tract with a cystoscope, for diagnostic and treatment purposes.

Cytogenetics: the science of chromosomes and genes.

Cytology: the science of cells.

Cytolysin: a substance able to dissolve living cells.

Cytoplasm: the portion of a living cell that surrounds the nucleus.

D

Darkfield examination: a test to diagnose syphilis during the first (primary) stage of the disease.

Normal values in fluid from the lesion: negative for Treponema organisms

---

Dehydroepiandrosterone: a sex hormone secreted by the testes and adrenal glands that stimulates development of secondary sex characteristics.

Normal values in urine after 24-hour collection: males—0.2-2.0 mg; females—0.2-1.8 mg

---

Delta-aminolevulinic acid: *see* δ-Aminolevulinic acid.

Deoxyribonucleic acid: a nucleic acid that is an essential component of a chromosome, and that carries the genetic information of the organism.

Diacetic acid: a ketone body produced in certain metabolic diseases such as uncontrolled diabetes; also known as acetoacetic acid.

Normal value in urine: negative

Diagnex Blue tubeless gastric analysis: a test done on urine to determine gastric acid secretion.

Normal value in urine: some free acid present

Dick test: a skin test to detect susceptibility to scarlet fever.

Normal value (not susceptible) in skin injected with scarlet fever toxin: negative (no skin reaction)

Differential blood count: a measurement of the percentages of the various types of leukocytes (white blood cells) in a sample of blood.

Normal values in whole blood:
neutrophils: 65% total, 58% mature, 7% young
lymphocytes: 27%
monocytes: 5%
eosinophils: 2%
basophils: 1%

Differential stain: a stain that allows distinction between various groups of microorganisms.

Dilatation and curettage: an operative procedure in which the cervix is dilated and a curette is passed into the uterus to obtain tissue specimens to diagnose a benign or malignant tumor or disease, to remove the products of conception, or for other purposes.

Diodrast clearance (in blood): the rate at which the kidneys remove Diodrast, an injected test substance, from the bloodstream; measured to evaluate kidney function.

Normal values in serum: 600-720 ml/minute

Diodrast clearance (in urine): rate at which the kidneys excrete Diodrast, an injected substance; tested to evaluate kidney function.

Normal values in timed urine: 600-720 ml/minute

Diplococci: a type of cocci (bacteria) found in pairs.

Discogram: radiographic record of an intervertebral disc (a round piece of cartilage separating spinal vertebrae) to diagnose such conditions as herniation.

Disinfectant: an agent that destroys disease-causing organisms and their products.

Disinfection: the use of a disinfectant to destroy disease-causing organisms and their products.

Droplet infection: infection acquired through the sneezing and coughing of another person.

Dysfunction: Abnormal or impaired function.

E

Echocardiogram: a scan of the heart using ultrasound to record the structure, position, and motion of the heart.

Echoencephalogram: a brain scan using ultrasound to detect such abnormalities as a tumor, clot, or hemorrhage.

Ectopic pregnancy: implantation of fertilized ovum outside the uterus.

Electroanalytical chemistry: a technique that utilizes the interaction of electricity with liquid to measure dissolved substances such as sodium, calcium, and potassium.

Electrocardiogram: a record of the heart's electrical activity and impulses via monitoring equipment and a printout strip; important in diagnosing abnormal heart rhythms.

Electroencephalogram: a record of the brain's electrical impulses and activity via monitoring equipment and a printout strip; important in studying epilepsy and other neurological conditions.

Electrolyte: a substance that conducts an electric current in solution.

Electromyogram: a record of electrical activity associated with muscle movement; done to evaluate muscle function and diagnose dysfunction.

Electrophoresis: a laboratory technique that involves the movement of suspended particles in an electrical field; useful for separating and identifying blood substances such as serum proteins, lipoproteins, isoenzymes, and hemoglobin types. *See also* Citrate agar hemoglobin electrophoresis.

Electrophoresis, protein: a method of determining the presence and quantity of proteins.

Normal values in serum:
albumin: 52-65%; 3.2-5.6 gm/dl
globulin:
  alpha-1: 2.5-5.0%; 0.1-0.4 gm/dl
  alpha-2: 7.0-13.0%; 0.4-1.2 gm/dl
  beta: 8.0-14.0%; 0.5-1.1 gm/dl
  gamma: 12.0-22.0%; 0.5-1.6 gm/dl

Normal values in cerebrospinal fluid:
pre-albumin: 4.1±1.2%
albumin: 62.4±5.6%
globulin:
  alpha-1: 5.3±1.2%
  alpha-2: 8.2±2.0%
  beta: 12.8±2.0%
  gamma: 7.2±1.1%

Embolism: blocking of a blood vessel by a clot or foreign material.

Emergency radiography: X-ray procedures done after a patient has been injured or developed signs of serious illness, often performed in the emergency department of a hospital.

Endocrine: ductless; refers to activities and hormonal secretions of ductless glands.

Endogenous: originating in a gland or other internal part of the body.

Endoscopy: examination of internal body areas (larynx, esophagus, stomach, uterus, rectum, colon) with an endoscope—a device consisting of a tube with a light, refracting mirrors, and other diagnostic and therapeutic accessories—for diagnosis and treatment. *See also* Fiberoptic endoscopy.

Endotoxin: a toxin liberated during the destruction of a bacterial or other microbial cell.

Enteric bacteria: bacteria that live in the gastrointestinal tract.

Enterotoxin: a toxin found in contaminated food that causes vomiting, diarrhea, and possibly serious gastrointestinal illness.

Enteroviruses: viruses that live in the gastrointestinal tract.

Enzyme: a protein substance secreted by body cells that can act as a catalyst—changing or modifying other body secretions and processes without being changed itself.

Epidemic: an infection that attacks large groups of people; it typically starts in one local area and is spread to larger segments of a population, sometimes to other countries or even worldwide.

Epidemiology: the science of tracking widespread contagious and other diseases.

Epinephrine: an adrenal hormone, somewhat elevated in certain psychiatric illnesses, and indicative of pheochromocytoma (a tumor of the adrenal gland) when sharply elevated.

Normal values in urine after 24-hour collection: 0-20 mcg

Epstein-Barr virus: a herpes virus, also believed to cause mononucleosis.

Erythrocyte: red blood cell.

Erythrocyte count: a count of erythrocytes in a blood sample.

Normal values in whole blood: males—4.6-6.2 million/mm^3; females—4.2-5.4 million/mm^3

Erythrocyte hemolysis test: a test of the susceptibility of red blood cells to hemolysis, an indication of blood levels of vitamin E, which may be deficient in anemias, infertility, and malnutrition.

Normal values in plasma: 0.5 mg/dl

Erythrocyte indices: measures of size and hemoglobin concentration of red blood cells.

Normal values:
mean corpuscular volume: 82-98 cubic microns (fluid)
mean corpuscular hemoglobin: 27-31 pg/dl
mean corpuscular hemoglobin concentration: 32-36%

Erythrocyte sedimentation rate: the rate at which erythrocytes settle in unclotted (freshly drawn) blood; an indication of the presence and degree of various inflammatory diseases and infections.

Normal values in whole blood:
men under 50: less than 15 mm/hour
men over 50: less than 20 mm/hour
women under 50: less than 20 mm/hour
women over 50: less than 30 mm/hour

Esophagoscopy: examination of the esophagus with a scope to detect injury, growths, or other abnormalities.

Estrogen receptor test: a test of whether a patient's cancer is stimulated by (responds to) estrogen, to determine whether hormonal treatment will be helpful.

Estrogens, fractionated: estrogenic hormones individually measured in urine.

Normal values in urine after 24-hour collection (nonpregnant, midcycle female):
estrone (E1): 2-25 mcg
estradiol (E2): 0-10 mcg
estriol (E3): 2-30 mcg

Estrogens, total: estrogenic hormones measured together in urine.

Normal values in urine after 24-hour collection:
males—5-18 mcg; females—ovulation, 28-100 mcg; luteal peak, 22-105 mcg; menses, 4-25 mcg; pregnancy, up to 45,000 mcg; postmenopause, 14-20 mcg

Ethosuximide: an anticonvulsant medication monitored in the plasma to determine steady-state levels (reached 4-7 days after treatment is started).

Therapeutic values: 40-100 mcg/ml

Etiocholanolone: a sex hormone secreted by the testes and adrenal glands.

Continued

Normal values in urine after 24-hour collection:
males—1.4-5.0 mg; females—0.8-4.0 mg

Etiology: cause, usually of a disease.

Exchange transfusion: the repetitive removal of small amounts of blood, followed by substitution of like amounts of blood from a number of donors, until a large portion of the body's blood has been replaced.

Excretory urogram: *see* Intravenous pyelogram.

Exotoxin: a poison secreted by disease-causing microorganisms into their environment, such as the host's body.

Extracellular: outside the cell.

Eye sonogram: a test using ultrasound to detect diseases of the eye.

F

Fahrenheit: a temperature scale on which the freezing point of water is 32°F and the boiling point of water is 212°F. One degree Fahrenheit (1°F) equals 5/9 of a degree Celsius (centigrade, C).

Fat, neutral (in blood): measurement of fats, such as triglycerides, in the blood.

Normal values in serum or plasma: 0-200 mg/dl

Fat, neutral (in feces): a test done on feces to check for digestive or pancreatic disturbances.

Normal values in 72-hour feces: 1-5% of dry matter

Fat, qualitative: a urine test for fat, present only in patients with kidney abnormalities.

Normal value in urine: negative

Fat, total (in feces): the fat content of the feces; measured to determine whether fat is being absorbed normally and to check for disease states causing abnormal fat levels, such as nontropical sprue or pancreatic disease.

Normal values in 72-hour feces: 0-25% of weight of specimen; average less than 6 gm/24 hours

---

Fatty acids, free: lipid derivatives measured in feces to determine a patient's ability to digest fats.

Normal values in feces: 5-13% of dry matter

Fatty acids, total: lipid derivatives, including saturated and unsaturated fatty acids, measured in serum when disturbances of fat metabolism are suspected.

Normal values in serum: 190-420 mg/dl

Fatty acids, total free: measurement of blood levels of lipid (fatty) fractions stored in adipose tissues.

Normal values in serum: 9-15 mM/liter

Normal values in plasma: 300-480 microEq/liter

Feces: stool, bowel movement, intestinal discharge.

Ferritin: a blood protein that contains iron; measured to determine the amount of iron stored in the bone marrow, and to diagnose the causes of anemia or unexplained weakness.

Normal values in serum: 200-400 ng/dl

Fiberoptic endoscopy: the use of an endoscope—a flexible tube able to bend light rays—to inspect the interior of a body cavity or organ. Because it bends light rays, the scope can be used to see around corners and other obstacles to diagnose the location and type of disease, and to perform operative and other therapeutic procedures. *See also* Endoscopy.

Fibrinogen: a protein involved in blood clotting.

Normal values in plasma: 200-400 mg/dl

Fixation of tissue: the preservation of body tissue in preservative solution in preparation for microscopic or other examination.

Flame photometry: a laboratory technique involving the use of electrical particles (cations and anions) and light measurements to measure such substances as sodium, potassium, and lithium.

Fluorescent eye stain: an eye test to detect injury or other abnormality in the cornea or to aid in fitting contact lenses.

Normal value: no evidence of dye remains after tears have passed over the area

---

Fluorescent treponemal antibody absorption test: a blood test for Treponema pallidum, the organism that causes syphilis.

Normal value in serum: negative

Fluoride: a fluorine compound excreted in urine if present in the system.

Normal values in urine after 24-hour collection: less than 1 mg

---

Fluorometry: a laboratory technique for measuring substances that become fluorescent in ultraviolet light or when exposed to strong radiant energy. It is used primarily when measuring in very small units such as micrograms or nanograms per milliliter, as occurs in tests for urinary estrogens and catecholamines.

Fluoroscopy: a radiographic technique used to study the functions of internal body structures by projection of images on a fluorescent screen.

Folate: a folic acid salt. Folate deficiency occurs with alcoholism, birth control pills, malnutrition, and certain types of anemia.

Normal values in serum: 5-25 ng/ml (bioassay)

Normal values in erythrocytes: 166-640 ng/ml (bioassay)

Folic acid: a vitamin needed to prevent anemia; deficiency may occur with alcoholism, birth control pills, malnutrition, and certain diseases. Deficiency is detected by measuring blood levels of folates.

Normal values in serum: 5-25 ng/ml (bioassay)

Follicle-stimulating hormone: a sex hormone that stimulates the development of egg and sperm cells.

Normal values in urine after 24-hour collection (female): adults—6-50 mouse uterine units (MUU); prepubertal—less than 10 MUU; postmenopausal—more than 50 MUU

Forced expiratory volume: *see under* Timed.

Formiminoglutamic acid: an intermediate product in histidine metabolism; elevated in the urine of patients with deficiency of vitamin B_{12} or folates.

Normal values in urine: less than 3 mg/24 hours; after taking 15 gm of L-histidine—4 mg/8 hours

Fragility test: *see* Osmotic fragility test.

Fructose: a natural sugar excreted in urine.

Normal values in urine after 24-hour collection: 30-65 mg

Fulminating infection: a sudden, overwhelming infection.

Fumigation: sterilization of an object or area by exposure to gas fumes.

Fungus: a microbic vegetable organism that subsists on molds and other living matter. Some fungi can cause disease.

G

Galactose: a milk sugar derivative.

Normal values in whole blood: adults—none; children—less than 20 mg/dl

---

Gallbladder series: a series of X-ray studies of the gallbladder and related structures; done after the patient swallows contrast medium that outlines the parts to be studied.

Gamma globulin: a blood protein fraction that contains antibodies.

Normal values in serum: 0.5-1.6 gm/dl

Gamma-glutamyl transpeptidase: *see* γ-Glutamyl transpeptidase.

Gastric analysis: analysis of fluid aspirated from the stomach to diagnose various diseases, or to determine the types and quantities of drugs ingested in an overdose.

Gastric fluid, basal acid output: a test to measure the total output of stomach acid in an hour, after the patient has been intubated.

Normal values: 0-6 mEq/hour

Gastric fluid, basal acid output/maximal acid output ratio: the ratio of basal to maximal acid output; if greater than normal, it may indicate various disease states of the stomach or intestines.

Normal values: less than 0.4

Gastric fluid, fasting residual volume: residual volume of gastric acid secretion after 12 hours of fasting.

Normal values: 20-100 ml

Gastric fluid, maximal acid output: measurement of stomach acid secretion following stimulation by injection of histamine. If maximal levels are elevated, anemia, stomach infection, or other stomach disease may be present.

Normal values: 5-40 mEq/hour

Gastric fluid, pH: a measure of the acidity or alkalinity of gastric fluid.

Gastrointestinal series: a series of X-ray studies of the esophagus, stomach, and small bowel; done after the patient swallows barium contrast medium to outline the parts to be studied.

Gastroscopy: examination of the stomach and upper gastrointestinal tract with a gastroscope.

Generalized infection: an infection that affects the entire body.

Genetic: carried by the genes; inherited.

Germ: a microbe that may cause disease.

Germicide: a substance that kills microbes.

Giemsa's stain: a solution used for staining microorganisms, such as protozoa, rickettsiae, and viral inclusion bodies, to make them detectable in laboratory samples.

GI series: *see* Gastrointestinal series.

Globulins: a group of blood proteins that are soluble in various weak salt solutions, but insoluble in water. Each type of globulin has a different biochemical function. *See* Electrophoresis, protein.

Globulins (in cerebrospinal fluid): measurement of globulin fraction in cerebrospinal fluid.

Normal values in CSF: qualitative—negative; quantitative—6-16 mg/dl

---

Globulins, total: measurement of blood levels of the entire group of globulins.

Normal values in serum: 2.3-3.5 gm/dl

Glucose (in cerebrospinal fluid): a natural sugar found in cerebrospinal fluid. CSF levels are measured to detect abnormal conditions of the spinal cord and brain. Levels are decreased in meningitis.

Normal values in CSF: 45-75 mg/dl

Glucose difference, synovial fluid-blood: *see under* Synovial fluid.

Glucose, fasting: measurement of blood sugar levels after a 12-hour fast; done to diagnose diabetes.

Normal values in serum or plasma: 70-110 mg/dl

Normal values in whole blood: 60-100 mg/dl

Glucose-6-phosphate dehydrogenase: a red blood cell enzyme; levels are decreased in a type of anemia.

Normal values in red blood cells: 250-500 units/10^9 cells; 1200-2000 mIU/ml of packed red cells

---

Glucose, qualitative: a urine test for glucose; present in metabolic diseases such as diabetes.

Normal values in urine: negative or trace

Glucose tolerance test (oral): a metabolic test in which a fasting patient drinks a quantity of glucose. Blood sugar levels are then measured at intervals of ½, one, two, three, and four hours.

Normal values in urine: negative or trace

Normal values in serum or plasma:
fasting: 70-110 mg/dl
at 30 minutes: 30-60 mg/dl above fasting level
at 60 minutes: 20-50 mg/dl above fasting level
at 120 minutes: 5-15 mg/dl above fasting level
at 180 minutes: fasting level or below

γ-Glutamyl transpeptidase: an enzyme elevated in the blood of heavy drinkers of alcoholic beverages.

Normal values in blood: less than 25 units per liter

Glutathione: an enzyme whose deficiency may lead to hemolytic anemia.

Normal values in whole blood: 24-37 mg/dl

Gonadotropins, pituitary: hormones secreted by the pituitary gland that stimulate the ovaries or testes. They include FSH and LH.

Normal values in urine after 24-hour collection (female):
10-50 mouse uterine units

Gram-negative microorganisms: those that do not retain the violet dye used in the Gram stain method, and take the color of the counterstain.

Gram-positive microorganisms: those that retain the violet dye used in the Gram stain method, and do not accept the counterstain.

Gram stain: a staining procedure used in the laboratory to distinguish between different types of microorganisms.

Grouping, typing: the classification of specific microbes, blood types, cells, or genetic components according to certain common characteristics.

Guaiac test: a test performed on feces or urine to detect occult blood in the intestinal or urinary tract. Guaiac, a wood resin, is the reagent used in the laboratory procedure.

Normal value in feces after 3 days of meat-free diet: negative

Normal value in urine: negative

Guanase: an enzyme found in the blood that is sometimes markedly elevated in patients with hepatitis and other types of liver disease, and in infectious mononucleosis.

Normal values in serum: less than 3 nanomols/ml/minute

Guthrie bacterial inhibition assay: a blood or urine test for phenylalanine, an amino acid with elevated levels in patients with phenylketonuria, an inherited enzyme deficiency disease that causes mental retardation if not diagnosed and treated soon after birth.

Normal values in blood: negative to trace

Normal value in urine: negative

H

Half-life: the length of time required for a given isotope's radioactivity to decay to half its original potency.

Haptoglobin: a blood protein that combines with hemoglobin; a low level indicates a breakdown of red blood cells, which may occur in certain diseases, snakebite, or drug ingestion. Levels are increased in some inflammatory conditions.

Normal values in serum: 50-200 mg/dl

HCG radioreceptor assay: a reliable, simple urine test to diagnose early pregnancy, ectopic pregnancy, and missed abortion. HCG (human chorionic gonadotropin) is found only in pregnancy or in HCG-producing tumors.

Normal values in urine: negative within 2 hours if the patient is not pregnant; positive within 1 hour if the patient is pregnant

---

Heart catheterization: a diagnostic procedure that involves inserting a catheter into a vein or artery and advancing it under fluoroscopic guidance into the blood vessels or chambers of the heart. Contrast medium is injected to aid in visualization, and blood samples and pressure readings may be taken at different stages.

Heart scan: a scan of the heart after injection of a radioactive substance into a vein, to determine size, shape, and location; to diagnose pericarditis (inflammation and fluid accumulation around the heart); or to view the heart's chambers. A blood pool scan can measure damage sustained after a heart attack.

Hematocrit: the relative volume of red blood cells in whole blood.

Normal values in venous blood: males—40-54%; females—38-47%

Hematogenous: originating or carried in the blood.

Hematology: the science of blood, blood-forming organs, and blood diseases.

Hematuria: blood in the urine.

Hemoglobin A_2: a type of hemoglobin accounting for 1.5-3.5% of normal adult hemoglobin; it is elevated in various blood diseases.

Normal values in blood: 1.5-3.5% of total hemoglobin

Hemoglobin (in blood): the oxygen-carrying protein pigment in red blood cells. *Continued*

Normal values in serum or plasma: qualitative—negative; quantitative: 0.5-5.0 mg/dl

Normal values in whole blood: females—12.0-16.0 gm/dl; males—13.5-18.0 gm/dl

---

Hemoglobin F: fetal hemoglobin; in adults or children, abnormally elevated levels may indicate various blood diseases and conditions, including aplastic anemia, leukemia, and thalassemia, a type of hemolytic anemia.

Normal values in blood: Hemoglobin F is the major constituent of fetal blood, but normally constitutes less than 2% of hemoglobin in adults.

Hemoglobin (in urine): the oxygen-carrying protein pigment in red blood cells; found in the urine only in the presence of an abnormality or disease of the genitourinary tract.

Normal value in urine: negative

Hemogram: a laboratory record, either written or graphic, of the differential blood count, with special emphasis on the size, shape, special characteristics, and numbers of the solid constituents of the blood. *See also* Complete blood count.

Hemolysis: the dissolving or destruction of red blood cells by a chemical substance or disease.

Hepatitis associated antigen (Australian antigen): an antigen often found in the serum of people who have had hepatitis; the blood test for this antigen is used to detect serum hepatitis (type B), and to differentiate it from type A hepatitis.

Normal value in serum: negative, but sometimes present in otherwise healthy Americans and in many people who live in the Middle East and Asia.

Herpes: a virus with several forms, capable of causing painful infection of lips, trunk, nerves, or genitals.

Heterophil antibody test: a test using sheep red blood cells to diagnose infectious mononucleosis.

Normal value in serum: titer of less than 1:56

Hinton test: a blood test for syphilis.

Normal value in serum: negative

Histoplasma agglutinins: agglutinins associated with fungal lung infection.

Normal values in serum: titer of less than 1:8

Homogentisic acid: an acid present in urine in alkaptonuria, a rare metabolic disease.

Normal value in urine: negative

Homovanillic acid: a product of normal metabolism; elevated urine levels may indicate various tumors of the adrenal gland.

Normal values in urine after 24-hour collection: less than 15 mg

---

Host: an animal or plant that supports a parasite.

Human chorionic gonadotropin: *see* HCG radioreceptor assay.

Human growth hormone: a hormone secreted by the pituitary gland. Blood levels provide a measure of pituitary function.

Normal values in serum: less than 10 ng/ml

Human leukocyte locus A antigen: a tissue antigen found on cell surfaces; important in establishing tissue compatibility in crossmatching prior to transplantation of an organ such as a kidney.

Human placental lactogen: a hormone secreted by the placenta during pregnancy; levels may be decreased in certain abnormalities of pregnancy.

Normal values in serum after 5th week of pregnancy: 0.5 mcg/ml, with gradual rise to 7-10 mcg/ml at time of delivery

---

Hydrocortisone: *see* Cortisol.

11-Hydroxyandrosterone: a sex hormone secreted by the testes and adrenal glands.

Normal values in urine after 24-hour collection: males—0.1-0.8 mg; females—0.0-0.5 mg

α-Hydroxybutyric dehydrogenase: an enzyme in blood that may be elevated after tissue damage, such as occurs in heart attack.

Normal values in serum: 140-350 U/ml

17-Hydroxycorticosteroids: a group of hormones, including cortisol and others, secreted by the cortex (outer layer) of the adrenal glands; urine levels are measured as a test of adrenal function and to diagnose hypo- or hyperadrenalism.

Normal values in urine after 24-hour collection: males—5.5-14.5 mcg; females—4.9-12.9 mcg; lower in children. After injection of 25 USP units ACTH, level is 2-4 times higher.

11-Hydroxyetiocholanolone: a sex hormone secreted by the testes and adrenal glands.

Normal values in urine after 24-hour collection: males—0.2-0.6 mg; females—0.1-1.1 mg

---

5-Hydroxyindoleacetic acid (in blood): an end product of serotonin metabolism. Serotonin normally constricts blood vessels and transmits nerve impulses, but also produces flushing, rapid heartbeat, asthma, diarrhea, and other symptoms when present in abnormally high levels, as in certain tumors.

Normal values as serotonin in whole blood:
0.05-0.20 mcg/ml

5-Hydroxyindoleacetic acid (in urine): an end product of serotonin metabolism, elevated in the urine of patients with carcinoid syndrome—a condition produced by a type of tumor found in the appendix or other parts of the lower intestinal tract, and sometimes in the lungs.

Normal values in urine after 24-hour collection: 1-5 mg

Hydroxyproline: an amino acid with elevated levels in the urine in bone disease and certain inherited conditions, such as Marfan's syndrome.

Normal values in urine after 24-hour collection: 10-75 mg

5-Hydroxytryptamine (serotonin): a substance in blood and tissues that constricts blood vessels and transmits nerve impulses; it is elevated in the urine in carcinoid syndrome—a condition produced by a type of tumor found in the appendix or lower intestinal tract, and sometimes in the lungs.

Normal values in urine: 0.05-0.20 mcg/ml

Hyperimmune: unusually rich in antibodies; having greater than usual degree of immunity.

Hypersensitivity (allergy): excessive sensitivity of tissues to substances or other stimuli inside or outside the body.

Hypertonic solution: one that has a higher osmotic pressure than a standard (reference) solution.

Hypotonic solution: one that has a lower osmotic pressure than a standard (reference) solution.

Hysterogram: radiographic record of the uterus after injection of contrast medium into the uterine cavity.

Hysterosalpingography: X-ray studies of the uterus and fallopian tubes after contrast medium is injected.

Hysteroscopy: a procedure that allows direct visual examination of the uterus with a tubular instrument (endoscope) for diagnostic or treatment purposes.

I

Image intensifier: electronic equipment used in X-ray studies that allows fluoroscopy to be performed with a lower dose of radiation, yet produces a brighter, more detailed image than is possible with a conventional fluoroscopy screen. The image intensifier also allows the use of closed-circuit television of the process being studied.

Immune: protected against a given infection or disease process.

Immune bodies: antibodies that fight infection or agents foreign to the body.

Immune globulin: a blood protein fraction that contains antibodies.

Immune serum: serum that has immune properties (contains antibodies).

Immunity: resistance to disease or infection.

Immunity, acquired: immunity achieved sometime after birth.

Immunity, active: long-term ability of the cells to protect the body against a new infection, as a result of vaccination that stimulates development of specific antibodies.

Immunity, passive: temporary immunity conferred by injection or ingestion of prepared material containing antibodies against a specific disease.

Immunodiffusion: a laboratory technique used to detect the type and quantity of a substance, such as an abnormal immunoglobulin, for which an antibody is available.

Immunoelectrodiffusion: a laboratory technique similar to immunodiffusion, but speeded up by applying an electric current during the process.

Immunoglobulins (Ig) A, D, E, G, and M: a family of blood protein fractions, each with one or more specific functions. IgA is protective against viral and bacterial infections, and may cause transfusion reactions. The functions of IgD are not yet understood, although IgD can be isolated. IgE has a prominent role in allergic reactions, such as asthma or skin rash. IgG and IgM fight infection.

Normal values in serum: IgA—50-250 mg/dl; IgD—0.5-3.0 ml/dl; IgE—0.01-0.04 mg/dl; IgG—800-1,600 mg/dl; IgM—40-120 mg/dl

---

Immunohematology: the study of antigen-antibody reactions and their effects on blood.

Immunology: the science of immunity.

Inclusion bodies: variously shaped bodies (particles) that occur in cells occupied by viruses.

Incompatibility: a state in which two substances cannot be mixed without one of them being changed or destroyed.

Incubation period: the time between exposure to infection and the first symptoms of illness.

Incubator: a cabinet heated to a constant temperature to allow cultures of bacteria to grow; or a temperature-regulated apparatus for premature babies.

Indican: a substance excreted in the urine. Elevated levels may indicate that the patient is on a high-protein diet or suffering from gastrointestinal disease.

Normal values in urine after 24-hour collection: 10-20 mg

Infection: a disease that results from invasion of the body by disease-causing microorganisms that multiply and produce injurious effects.

Infectious: pertaining to an infection that can be transmitted.

Infiltrate: a foreign substance introduced in tissue.

Inflammation: tissue reaction to an injury or irritant; symptoms include redness, heat, and pain.

Inoculation: the introduction of infectious material or microbes into the body, usually to stimulate the development of immunity.

Insulin: a protein hormone secreted by the pancreas that regulates carbohydrate metabolism.

Normal values in serum after 12-hour fast: 5-30 microU/ml

Normal values in serum after glucose is administered: insulin level rises to above 200 microU/ml within 1 hour, then returns to normal within 4 hours. (This test cannot be done on a patient receiving insulin injections for treatment of diabetes.)

Intercurrent infection: one that develops in a person who already has another disease or infection.

Intravascular coagulation test: a test to detect internal coagulation of blood, a phenomenon that occurs in a number of blood coagulation disorders.

Normal value in whole blood: none

Intravenous pyelogram: radiographic record of the kidneys and urinary tract after intravenous injection of contrast medium to aid in visualization.

Intrinsic factor: *see* Unsaturated vitamin B_{12} binding capacity.

Inulin: a vegetable starch used in tests of kidney function.

Inulin clearance: the rate at which the kidneys excrete inulin; tested to evaluate kidney function and diagnose muscle or liver diseases.

Normal values in urine: 100-150 ml/minute

Iodine, butanol-extractable: iodine that can be separated from the plasma proteins by solvents such as butanol; it can be used as a measure of thyroid hormone levels in the blood to assess thyroid function.

Normal values in serum: 3.5-6.5 mcg/dl (results inaccurate if other forms of iodine given previously)

Iron-binding capacity: a measure of the iron uptake and return in blood, in relation to the synthesis and breakdown of hemoglobin.

Normal values in serum: 250-450 mcg/dl

Iron saturation, percent: the capacity of iron to saturate transferrin (an iron-binding substance); a measure of iron excess or deficiency.

Normal values in serum: 20-55%

Iron, total: measure of the total blood level of iron.

Normal values in serum: 50-150 mcg/dl

Isoantigen: an antigen that incites antibody production in members of the same species.

Isocitric dehydrogenase: an enzyme elevated in liver disease or placental problems of pregnancy.

Normal values in serum: 50-300 units/ml

Isoenzymes: enzymes with slightly different chemical structures, but producing the same effects.

Isotonic solution: one that has the same osmotic pressure as a standard (reference) solution.

Isotope: one of a variety of forms in which a chemical element can appear. Isotopes of an element are identical in number of protons and electrons in each atom, but differ in mass number (total number of protons and neutrons in each atom's nucleus), and therefore have different properties.

J

Jaundice: a state in which the skin and other body parts turn yellowish due to elevated blood levels of bilirubin.

K

Karyotyping: analysis of chromosomes; performed on fetal cells obtained by amniocentesis to detect the sex and various genetic factors or diseases of the unborn child. Karyotyping is also performed on children and young adults to detect genetic abnormalities and diseases.

11-Ketoandrosterone: a sex hormone secreted by the testes and adrenal glands.

Normal values in urine after 24-hour collection:
males—0.2-1.0 mg; females—0.2-0.8 mg

11-Ketoetiocholanolone: a sex hormone secreted by the testes and adrenal glands.

Normal values in urine after 24-hour collection:
males—0.2-1.0 mg; females—0.2-0.8 mg

Ketone bodies (in blood): a group of compounds produced by fatty acid metabolism, found only when a metabolic disturbance is present.

Normal value in serum: negative

Ketone bodies (in urine): a group of compounds produced by fatty acid metabolism, found only when a metabolic disturbance is present.

Normal value in urine: negative

17-Ketosteroids (in blood): a group of adrenal cortical hormones with altered blood levels in Addison's disease, Cushing's syndrome, stress, and endocrine disorders associated with precocious puberty, feminization in men, and excessive hair growth.

Normal values in plasma: less than 30 mcg/dl in the morning; less than 10 mcg/dl in the evening

17-Ketosteroids (in urine): a group of adrenal cortical hormones with altered urine levels in Addison's disease, Cushing's syndrome, stress, and endocrine disorders associated with precocious puberty, feminization in men, and excessive hair growth.

Normal values in urine after 24-hour collection: males—8-15 mg; females—6-11.5 mg; children, 12-15 yrs—5-12 mg; children under 12 yrs—less than 5 mg; levels increase 50-100% after injection of ACTH.

Knee endoscopy: the use of an endoscope to inspect the interior of the knee joint, to diagnose a torn cartilage or other abnormality. *See also* Arthroscopy.

Kolmer's test: a blood test for syphilis.

Normal value in serum: negative

Kymography: a technique used to record graphically the motions of body organs, such as the heart, and the great blood vessels.

L

Lactic acid: a monobasic acid, the end product of the metabolism of sugar. Blood levels of lactic acid are elevated in patients with lactic acidosis, diabetes, anemia, leukemia, following excessive exercise, and in other abnormal conditions.

Normal values in whole blood: venous—5-20 mg/dl; arterial—3-7 mg/dl

---

Lactic dehydrogenase (in blood): an enzyme in blood and tissues, elevated in various diseases, including myocardial infarction, cancer, and anemia.

Normal values in serum: 200-600 units/ml, or up to 250 IU/ml

Lactic dehydrogenase (in cerebrospinal fluid): an enzyme elevated in CSF in various conditions, including stroke and meningitis.

Normal values in CSF: approximately 1/10 of serum level

Lactic dehydrogenase isoenzymes: a variety of molecular forms of lactic dehydrogenase; the pattern of distribution of the various isoenzymes can help diagnose heart and liver disease.

Normal values in serum (separated by electrophoresis): anode—LDH_1 17-27%; LDH_2 27-37%; LDH_3 3-8%; LDH_4 0-5%; cathode—LDH_5 0-5%

Lactose: a sugar excreted in urine. Its levels are elevated in late pregnancy, during lactation, and in certain rare metabolic diseases.

Normal values in urine after 24-hour collection: 12-40 mg

Lactose tolerance: the capacity of the body to handle lactose/glucose metabolism.

Normal values in serum following ingestion of lactose: serum glucose changes are measured, and are comparable to those seen in a glucose tolerance test

Laryngoscopy: examination of the larynx and the upper portion of the trachea with a laryngoscope to diagnose a tumor or other abnormality or to remove a foreign body.

Latex fixation test: a blood test to detect various antibodies and factors indicative of such conditions as rheumatoid arthritis, lupus erythematosus, dermatomyositis, and chronic infections.

Normal value in serum: negative

Lead (in blood): a metallic element and normal blood constituent. If blood levels are elevated, lead poisoning is likely.

Normal values in whole blood: 0-5 mcg/dl

Lead (in urine): a metallic element that can be toxic if ingested; urine levels are elevated in patients with lead poisoning.

Normal values in urine after 24-hour collection:
less than 100 mcg

Lead apron, lead shield: a protective apron or device made of lead, worn by X-ray technicians, radiologists, and patients as protection against radiation during X-ray procedures.

Lecithin/sphingomyelin ratio: the ratio of two components of amniotic fluid; found to be a predictor of fetal lung maturity.

Normal value in AF: titer of 2:1 or greater

Leptospira agglutinins: agglutinins found in blood of patients with Weil's disease, an infectious type of jaundice caused by the Leptospira organism.

Normal value in serum: negative

Leukapheresis: a process in which blood is withdrawn from a vein, white blood cells are selectively removed in a cell separating machine, and the remainder of the blood is reinfused in the donor. The white blood cells may be used for treatment, research, or other purposes.

Leukocyte alkaline phosphatase test: a blood test done to detect various diseases that stimulate the secretion of this enzyme, such as cirrhosis, polycythemia, and certain infections. It is also used to differentiate chronic myelogenous leukemia from leukemoid reactions. (Test also known as neutrophil alkaline phosphatase test.)

Normal values in smear of fresh venous blood:
50-150 units

Lipase: a pancreatic enzyme active in fat digestion. It may be elevated in pancreatitis.

Normal values in serum: 0-1.5 Cherry-Crandall U/ml; 14-280 mIU/ml

---

Lipids: fatty acid fractions found in blood; elevated in certain diseases such as atherosclerosis.

Normal values in serum:
total: 400-800 mg/dl
cholesterol: 150-250 mg/dl
triglycerides: 10-190 mg/dl
fatty acids: 9.0-15.0 mM/liter
phospholipid as phosphorus: 9-16 mg/dl
phospholipids: 150-380 mg/dl
neutral fat: 0-200 mg/dl

Lithium: a metallic element; lithium compounds are used to treat certain types of mental illness. Lithium blood levels must be carefully monitored during treatment to avoid toxicity.

Continued

Normal values in serum: negative; therapeutic levels—0.5-1.5 mEq/liter

---

Liver scan: a scan of the liver after intravenous injection of a radioactive substance, to detect tumor, abscess, or degeneration, shown by a lack of uptake of the radioactive substance.

Long-acting thyroid-stimulating hormone: an agent with a prolonged effect on the thyroid gland; found in the blood in various thyroid conditions.

Normal value in serum: negative

Lumbar puncture: aspiration of fluid from the spinal canal through a needle, to diagnose stroke, infection, tumor, or other conditions, or to determine the extent of injury after head, neck, or back trauma.

Lung scan: (1) *Perfusion scan*—a scanning procedure involving intravenous injection of radioactive albumin and examination of lung structure and function, to diagnose pulmonary embolism. (2) *Ventilation scan*—a procedure in which the patient breathes in radioactive gas and the lungs are scanned for areas that don't receive air, or for other abnormalities.

Luteinizing hormone: a hormone that originates in the anterior portion of the pituitary gland and controls various reproductive functions.

Continued

Normal values in plasma: males—less than 11 mIU/ml; females—premenopausal, less than 25 mIU/ml; midcycle peak, more than 3 X baseline value; postmenopausal, more than 25 mIU/ml

---

Lymph: fluid that collects in body tissues, then flows through lymph glands and lymphatic channels into the venous circulation.

Lymphangiography: X-ray studies of lymph glands and lymphatic channels after injection of contrast medium.

M

Macroglobulins, total: heavy serum globulins, elevated in diseases including cancer and infections.

Normal values in serum: 70-430 mg/dl

Macroscopic: visible to the naked eye.

Magnesium: an essential mineral; measured in urine to detect deficiency or excess. Deficiency may indicate malnutrition, glandular hyperactivity, or other abnormalities. Excess levels may indicate dehydration, or inadequate adrenal function.

Normal values in urine after 24-hour collection:
6.0-8.5 mEq

Mammography: X-ray technique used to examine breast tissue for tumors or other abnormalities, and to differentiate between benign and malignant growths.

Mantoux test: a skin test to detect the presence of, or exposure to, tuberculosis.

Normal value: negative reaction if there is no disease or exposure

---

Mass spectrometry: an ionizing technique that uses the mass of compounds to identify and quantitate them. Peptides, catecholamines, bile acids, and various drugs are analyzed by this method.

Maximal acid output: *see under* Gastric fluid.

Maximum breathing capacity: the amount of air per minute a person can breathe.

Maximum midexpiratory flow: liters per second of air expelled during forced exhalation; a test of air flow obstruction.

Mazzini's test: a blood test for syphilis.

Normal value in serum: negative

Mean corpuscular hemoglobin: a measure of the average hemoglobin content per red blood cell.

Normal values in whole blood: 27-31 pg/cell

Mean corpuscular hemoglobin concentration: a measure of hemoglobin concentration in the average red blood cell; expressed as a ratio of hemoglobin to volume of packed red cells.

Normal values in whole blood: 32-36 gm/dl of packed red blood cells

Mean corpuscular volume: a measure of the average size of the red blood cells.

Normal values in whole blood: 82-98 cubic microns

Melanin, qualitative: a urine test for melanin, a normal pigment found in urine in malignant melanoma, a type of cancer.

Normal value in urine: negative

Metabolism: the physical and chemical changes in the body that are responsible for maintaining function and nutrition.

Metabolite: a product of metabolism.

Methemoglobin: a compound found in the blood following ingestion of nitrates, aspirin substitutes, and food preservatives.

Normal value in whole blood: negative

3-Methoxy-4-hydroxymandelic acid: an excretory product of the catecholamines (adrenaline and noradrenaline); tested in urine as an indirect measure of catecholamine levels. Elevated levels may raise the blood pressure, or indicate the presence of adrenal gland or nervous tissue tumors, and such conditions as muscular dystrophy and myasthenia gravis. Certain drugs, foods, stress, and exercise can also cause elevated levels.

Normal values in urine after 24-hour collection:
adults—1.5-7.5 mg; infants—83 mcg/kg of body weight

Microbe: a microscopic organism.

Microscopic: invisible without use of microscope.

Microsomal antibody: *see under* Thyroid.

Midstream catch urine specimen: a urine specimen collected during the middle of the flow of urine, after the urinary opening has been carefully cleaned.

Minimal inhibitory concentration or minimal bactericidal concentration: the lowest concentration in blood at which an antibiotic medication is effective against an infection. Venous blood, containing the infectious organism, is placed in a sterile tube and then inoculated into a liquid culture medium that contains several concentrations of antibiotic drug ranging from 100 mcg/ml to as low as 0.195 mcg/ml. The lowest concentration at which growth is arrested or the microorganism is killed is then reported, and this concentration is used to monitor further antibiotic treatment.

Minnesota Multiphasic Personality Inventory: a test consisting of 550 statements to be interpreted by the subject; used in clinical psychology for overall personality evaluation, and to determine the presence of various personality disorders, such as depression and schizophrenia.

Mixed culture: a culture that contains two or more different strains of organisms.

Monoamine oxidase: an enzyme that is inhibited by a group of drugs that are effective in the treatment of depression.

Morbidity: the state of being ill.

Mucus (in feces): a translucent, gelatinous material, normally present in feces in small quantities, but indicating bowel abnormality when present in larger quantities.

Normal values in stool: negative or small amount

Mycophage: a fungal virus.

Mycosis: any disease caused by a fungus.

Mycotoxin: a toxin produced by fungi.

Myelography: X-ray studies of the spinal cord after injection of contrast medium.

Myoglobin: an oxygen-carrying protein normally present in muscle tissue; found in urine when there is extensive muscle destruction.

Normal values in urine after 24-hour collection: qualitative—negative; quantitative: less than 1.5 mg/liter

N

Needle biopsy: a sample of body tissue or fluid obtained via aspiration with a syringe and needle.

Neuroradiology: X-ray studies of the central nervous system, including brain and spinal cord.

Neutral fat: *see under* Fat.

Nitrogen, total (in feces): the nitrogen content of the feces; measured to detect such conditions as pancreatic insufficiency or impaired protein digestion.

Normal values in 24-hour specimen: 10% of intake, or 1-2 gm

Nonprotein nitrogen: the nitrogen in the blood not appearing as protein; about half is normally present as urea. Blood levels can be measured to determine kidney function.

Normal values in serum or plasma: 20-35 mg/dl

Normal values in whole blood: 25-50 mg/dl

Nosocomial infection: an infection acquired by a patient while in the hospital.

Nuclear medicine: a branch of medicine that uses radioisotopes in diagnostic and treatment procedures.

Nuclear scanning (radionuclide organ imaging): a diagnostic procedure in which a radioactive substance (radioisotope or radionuclide) is administered orally or by injection. A scanning device is then used to detect radioactivity over particular body areas. The size, shape, location, and function of body parts can then be recorded via a computer printout. The radioactive materials used do not harm the patient.

Nucleic acids: chemical compounds, found in all living cells, that are responsible for the transmission of hereditary characteristics.

Nucleolus: a spherical body inside the cell's nucleus that participates in the multiplication and metabolism of the cell.

5'-Nucleotidase: a nonlipid enzyme, elevated in some liver diseases, used to distinguish between certain liver and bone diseases.

Normal values in serum: 0-1.6 units

Nucleus: the central body of the cell that determines its functions.

O

Occult: hidden; obscure.

Occult blood: *see* Blood, occult.

Operating room radiography: X-ray studies carried out in the operating room during a surgical procedure.

Ophthalmoscopy: a direct, visual examination of the interior structures of the eye with an ophthalmoscope, for diagnostic or other purposes.

Opsonins: blood components that enable cells to fight off microorganisms that invade the body.

Ornithine carbamoyl transferase: an enzyme found in the blood in increased levels in liver and other diseases.

Normal values in serum: 8-20 mIU/ml

Osmolality, blood: the osmotic concentration of blood; a measure of its physicochemical properties.

Normal values in serum: 280-295 mOsm/liter

Osmolality, urine: the osmotic concentration of urine.

Normal values in urine: 500-800 mOsm/liter

Osmosis: the process by which fluid passes across a permeable membrane from a solution of lesser, to a solution of greater concentration.

Osmotic fragility test: a blood test in which red cells are placed in a series of successively weaker salt solutions to detect the point at which hemolysis (breakdown of red cells) occurs from osmotic pressure difference. Abnormally fragile cells break down in stronger solutions.

Normal values in 24 hours at 37° C: Hemolysis begins in 0.45 to 0.39% salt solution, and is complete in 0.33 to 0.30% salt solution

Ova and parasites test: microscopic examination of feces for parasites such as worms or amebae and their eggs (ova), to detect parasitic infection.

Oxygen: a gas forming about 21% of atmospheric air; essential to respiration.

Normal values in arterial whole blood: partial pressure (pO_2)—95-100 mm Hg; capacity—16-24 vol%; content—15-23 vol%; saturation: 94-100% of capacity

P

Pacemaker, artificial: a device that provides electrical stimulation to regulate the heartbeat.

Pacemaker installation fluoroscopy: fluoroscopic monitoring used to guide the insertion of a pacemaker.

Pancreas scan: a scan of the pancreas after intravenous injection of a radioactive substance, to diagnose a tumor, cyst, infection, or other abnormality.

Pandemic: an epidemic disease that affects a large area, possibly one or more entire continents.

Pap (Papanicolaou) smear: microscopic examination of cells taken from different parts of the body, often the cervix and vagina, to detect abnormalities such as cancer, infection, and effects of irradiation, and to determine cellular hormonal activity.

Para-aminohippuric acid, sodium (clearance): rate at which the kidneys remove this substance from the blood; measured to detect kidney damage or certain muscle diseases.

Normal values: in serum—600-750 ml/minute;
in urine (24-hour specimen)—600-750 ml/minute

Paracentesis: the puncture and withdrawal of fluid from the abdominal cavity, usually to remove excessive fluid accumulated by a disease process.

Parasite: an organism that survives by feeding on another.

Partial pressure of carbon dioxide: the portion of total gas pressure exerted by the carbon dioxide in blood; increased in certain respiratory conditions and in chest injuries; decreased in uncontrolled diabetes, liver or kidney disease, severe diarrhea, and during rapid breathing.

Normal values in arterial blood: 35-45 mm Hg

Normal values in venous blood: 40-45 mm Hg

Partial pressure of oxygen: the portion of total gas pressure exerted by oxygen in its gas phase in equilibrium with blood; decreased in obstructive lung disease, asthma, heavy exercise, and certain blood diseases.

Normal values in arterial blood: 95-100 mm Hg

Partial thromboplastin time: a blood test to screen for coagulation (clotting) disorders such as hemophilia, or to monitor anticoagulant medication.

Normal values in plasma: 60-85 seconds (after addition of partial thromboplastin reagent and ionized calcium)

Passive immunity: temporary immunity conferred by injection or ingestion of prepared material containing antibodies against a specific disease.

Patch test: a skin test for sensitivity to a particular substance. A small amount of solution containing the substance in question is placed on the patient's arm and covered, and the skin is observed for a reaction a few days later.

Reaction evaluation: considered positive if the skin area becomes red, swollen, irritated, or develops blisters

Pathology: the science of disease.

Paul-Bunnell test: a blood test for heterophil antibodies, used to confirm the diagnosis of infectious mononucleosis. *See also* Heterophil antibody test.

Normal value: negative

Pelvimetry: manual measurement or X-ray studies of the pelvic bones to determine if the space is adequate for giving birth.

Pentose: a type of sugar, elevated after ingestion of plums and cherries, and in certain rare diseases.

Normal values in urine after 24-hour collection: 2-5 mg/kg

Percutaneous transhepatic cholangiography: an X-ray technique in which dye is injected through the liver into the bile duct to detect obstruction.

Perfusion scan: *see* Lung scan.

Peripheral arteriovenography: X-ray studies of the arteries and veins in the peripheral parts of the body, such as the arms and legs, following injection of contrast medium into a peripheral artery or vein.

Petri dish: a covered glass dish used in the laboratory to grow microorganisms.

---

pH: the degree of acidity or alkalinity of a substance. The neutral point is pH 7; values below 7 indicate acidity; values above 7 indicate alkalinity. Maximum acidity is pH 0; maximum alkalinity is pH 14.

---

pH, blood: the hydrogen ion concentration (acidity or alkalinity) of blood.

Normal values in whole blood: arterial—7.38-7.44; venous—7.36-7.41

Normal values in venous serum or plasma: 7.35-7.45

---

pH, urine: the hydrogen ion concentration (acidity or alkalinity) of urine.

Normal values in urine: 4.6-8.0

Phage typing: identification of bacteria by testing their susceptibility to bacterial viruses.

Phagocyte: a cell that consumes bacteria and other foreign matter.

Phenobarbital/phenytoin serum levels: the concentrations of these drugs in the serum; monitored to maintain blood levels adequate to control seizures but not high enough to cause toxic reactions.

Therapeutic values: 10-30 mcg of each drug per milliliter of whole blood

Phenol coefficient: a measure of disinfectant activity of a given chemical in relation to carbolic acid (phenol).

Phenolsulfonphthalein: a dye used in kidney function tests. Urine levels are measured at regular intervals after injection of 6 mg, to test the excretory capacity of the kidney tubules. Rate of excretion is decreased in kidney and some urinary tract diseases, increased in some liver diseases.

Normal values in urine:
after 15 minutes—20-50% of dye excreted;
after 30 minutes—16-24%;
after 60 minutes—9-17%;
after 120 minutes—3-10%

Phenylalanine: an amino acid that accumulates in excessive amounts in phenylketonuria, an inherited enzyme deficiency disease that causes mental retardation if not diagnosed and treated soon after birth.

Normal values in serum: adults—less than 3.0 mg/dl; newborns (term)—1.2-3.5 mg/dl

Phenylpyruvic acid: an intermediate product of phenylalanine metabolism; present in the urine in certain metabolic diseases of the newborn.

Normal values in urine (qualitative): negative

Phenylketonuria: *see* Phenylalanine; Guthrie bacterial inhibition assay.

Phonocardiography: a procedure in which a transducer is applied to the chest to identify abnormal heart sounds in such conditions as heart valve disease and heart enlargement; frequently done in combination with apexcardiography and electrocardiography.

Phosphatase, acid (total): an enzyme present in kidney, serum, semen, and the prostate gland; increased in serum in trauma or cancer of the prostate, and various other conditions; also used to screen for the presence of semen in rape cases.

Normal values in serum: 0-1.1 Bodansky units/ml

Phosphatase, alkaline (total): an enzyme present in teeth, bone, plasma, kidney, and intestine; increased in serum in certain bone, liver, and other diseases.

Normal values in serum: adults—1.5-4.5 Bodansky units/dl; children—5.0-14.0 Bodansky units/dl

---

Phosphatase, leukocyte alkaline: *see under* Leukocyte.

Phosphorus, inorganic: phosphorus measured in the blood as phosphate ions. Elevated levels may indicate kidney, bone, and glandular diseases. Lowered levels may indicate alcoholism, vitamin deficiency, and other disease states.

Normal values in serum: adults—1.8-2.6 mEq/liter; children—2.3-4.1 mEq/liter

---

Phosphorus (in urine): a mineral essential to normal body function. Abnormal urine levels may indicate kidney, liver, bone, and other diseases.

Normal values in urine after 24-hour collection: 0.9-1.3 gm (may vary with intake)

Photometry: *see under* Flame.

Photoscan: a map of the distribution of a radiopharmaceutical in the body.

Phytohemagglutinin test: a test to detect genetic carriers of cystic fibrosis, an inherited disease that affects the sweat glands and lungs.

Normal value in white blood cells: a noticeable increase in cell protein when exposed to phytohemagglutinin

Pinocytosis: the process whereby cells take in fluids.

Pirquet's test: a skin test to detect the presence of, or exposure to, tuberculosis.

Placental scan: a scanning procedure performed on a pregnant woman after intravenous injection of a radioactive substance to locate the fetus and placenta and detect intrauterine bleeding, which would require immediate treatment.

Plasma: the fluid portion of the blood, including fibrinogen; as distinguished from serum, from which fibrinogen has been separated.

Plasmapheresis: a process in which blood is temporarily withdrawn from a donor via a closed system, the plasma is separated out, and the remaining blood components are returned; used to obtain blood fractions for patients deficient in them, or to treat disease conditions in the donor.

Plasma renin activity: the action of renin, an enzyme secreted by the kidney that influences salt and water balance; measured to detect adrenal disease associated with high blood pressure, and to evaluate various predictive factors concerning treatment.

Normal values in plasma: 0.2-4.0 ng/ml/hour (varies with salt intake and length of time in upright position prior to test)

Plasma volume: measurement of total volume of plasma; elevated in liver and spleen disease and vitamin C deficiency, decreased in dehydration, shock, and Addison's disease.

Normal values in whole blood: males—39 ml/kg; females—40 ml/kg

---

Platelet count: the number of platelets (thrombocytes) in a sample of blood. Platelets, essential in blood clotting, may be reduced in number in some blood diseases and after chemotherapy.

Normal values in whole blood: 150,000-400,000/microliter

Pneumoencephalography: X-ray studies of fluid-containing structures of the brain, using sterile gas injected into the spinal cord as contrast medium.

Porphobilinogen: a compound present in the urine in porphyria, a congenital metabolic disease.

Normal values in urine after 24-hour collection: qualitative—negative; quantitative—0-2.0 mg

---

Portable radiography: X-ray studies performed at the patient's bedside with portable X-ray equipment.

Postoperative radiography: X-ray studies performed immediately after an operation, in the recovery room, intensive-care unit, or patient's room.

Potassium (in blood): an essential electrolyte that regulates heart muscle activity, cellular fluid balance, and various enzyme reactions.

Normal values in plasma: 3.8-5.0 mEq/liter

Potassium (in urine): an essential electrolyte that regulates heart muscle activity, cellular fluid balance, and various enzyme reactions.

Normal values in urine after 24-hour collection:
40-80 mEq (can vary with diet)

PPD test: *see* Purified protein derivative test.

Precipitins: antibodies that are capable of reacting with specific soluble antigens to cause precipitation (clumping).

Pregnancy test: *see* HCG radioreceptor assay.

Pregnanediol: a metabolic product of progesterone; elevated in the urine of women during pregnancy and cyclically with the menstrual cycle; measured to detect ovulation, placental dysfunction, and feminization syndrome in men.

Normal values in urine after 24-hour collection: males—0-1 mg; females—premenopause, 1-8 mg (peak at 1 week after ovulation); pregnancy, 60-100 mg; postmenopause, 0.2-1.0 mg; children—negative

---

Pregnanetriol: a progesterone derivative; elevated in adrenogenital disease and Cushing's syndrome.

Normal values in urine after 24-hour collection: males—1.0-2.0 mg; females—0.5-2.0 mg; children—less than 0.5 mg

---

Preservative: an agent that is added to fluid (as in food or medicine)' that prevents the growth of microbial organisms.

Procainamide (Pronestyl): a drug used to control irregular or abnormal heart rhythms; monitored to maintain blood levels adequate to control heart rhythm but not high enough to cause toxic reactions.

Therapeutic values in whole blood drawn 4-6 hours after the most recent dose: 4-8 mcg/ml

---

Proctoscopy: direct examination of the anus and rectum with a proctoscope, to detect abnormalities.

Proctosigmoidoscopy: direct examination of the rectum and sigmoid colon with a scope.

Progesterone receptor test: a test of a tumor's response to progesterone, to predict whether the tumor is likely to respond to hormonal therapy.

Prolactin (lactogenic hormone): a pituitary hormone that stimulates milk secretion; measured in new mothers with lactation problems, women with menstrual problems, or when brain tumor is suspected.

Normal values in serum: 5-25 ng/ml; higher during pregnancy and lactation

Propranolol (Inderal): a medication used to reduce high blood pressure, slow the heart rate, treat angina pectoris, and prevent migraine headache; monitored in the blood to maintain levels that are therapeutically adequate but not high enough to cause toxic reactions.

Therapeutic values in whole blood, drawn 4 hours after the last dose or just before the upcoming dose: 50-120 mcg/ml

Protein (in blood): nitrogenous compounds, essential in tissue growth and repair; abnormal blood levels may indicate kidney, liver, and other diseases.

Normal values in serum: total—6.0-7.8 gm/dl; albumin—3.2-5.6 gm/dl (52-65% of total); globulin—2.3-3.5 gm/dl (38-44% of total)

Protein-bound iodine: iodine chemically bound to protein in the serum; measured as a test of thyroid function.

Normal values in serum: 4.0-8.0 mcg/dl (test results inaccurate if other forms of iodine given previously)

Protein (in cerebrospinal fluid): measurement of total CSF protein to detect such conditions as inflammation of the brain or spinal cord, or brain hemorrhage.

Normal values in CSF: lumbar—15-45 mg/dl; ventricular—8-15 mg/dl

Protein electrophoresis: *see* Electrophoresis.

Protein (in urine): measurement of urine protein to detect kidney disease.

Normal values in urine after 24-hour collection: qualitative—negative; quantitative—10-100 mg

Prothrombin consumption test: a test of one of the phases in the blood clotting process; a measure of the blood's ability to generate a normal amount of thromboplastin.

Normal values in serum: more than 80% consumption of prothrombin from the serum within 15 seconds or more, measured 1 hour after coagulation.

Prothrombin time: time required for clot formation in plasma; a measure of the activity of several coagulation factors.

Normal values in plasma: 12-14 seconds

Protoplasm: living matter; the essential substance of which cells are made, composed mainly of nucleic acids, proteins, lipids, carbohydrates, and inorganic salts.

Protoporphyrin: an important natural compound that occurs as an iron complex in hemoglobin and other blood pigments. Elevated levels indicate porphyria (a congenital metabolic disease), lead poisoning, liver disease, or certain cancers.

Normal values in red blood cells: 15-50 mcg/dl

Pulmonary arteriography: X-ray studies of the pulmonary arteries and related blood vessel structures after injection of contrast medium.

Purified protein derivative test: a skin test to detect susceptibility or exposure to tuberculosis.

Pus (in feces): a test to detect infection in the intestinal tract.

Normal value in feces: negative

Pyelography: X-ray studies of the kidneys and urinary tract after injection of contrast medium, to diagnose abnormalities or disease.

Pyruvate: a substance in blood; deficiency causes anemia.

Normal values in whole blood: 0.3-0.9 mg/dl

Q

Quantity not sufficient: terminology used for lab specimen submitted in an amount too small to be examined; the report is labeled QNS and returned.

Quantitative radiocardiography: a noninvasive radiological procedure that measures the flow of blood through the heart and lungs; it can be used as a screening test in healthy patients or for those with heart disease or other conditions.

R

RAD (radiation absorbed dose): a unit of radiation exposure that measures the absorbed dose.

Radarkymography: a noninvasive procedure that shows the size and outline of the heart; electrical impulses are passed over the surface of the chest, picked up by radar tracking equipment, and projected on a fluoroscopic screen.

Radiation therapy: treatment by X-rays or other forms of radiation; used in cancer and other diseases.

Radioactive decay: the loss of radioactive energy.

Radioactive iodine uptake: a test for thyroid disorders; the thyroid's absorption of oral or intravenous radioactive iodine is measured with a scintillation counter at 1, 6, or 24 hours after ingestion.

Normal values: 9-19% in 1 hour; 7.5-25% in 6 hours; 10-50% in 24 hours

---

Radioactivity: the breaking down of atomic nuclei, causing release of alpha, beta, or gamma rays.

Radioallergosorbent assay test: *see* Radioimmunosorbent assay test.

Radiography: the use of X-rays or other forms of radiation to produce an image of a body part.

Radioimmunoassay: a laboratory technique using a radioactive-labeled agent to measure antigens, antibodies, and other proteins in blood plasma.

Radioimmunosorbent assay test: a test using serum immunoglobulin E to detect allergic reactions to environmental substances such as animal hair, grasses, cosmetics, and dust.

Normal value in serum: negative

Radioisotope: an isotope that is radioactive; radioisotopes are used clinically in diagnostic and therapeutic procedures.

Radionuclide: a type of radioactive substance made up of atoms that disintegrate, emitting electromagnetic radiation.

Radionuclide angiocardiography: radiographic examination of the blood vessels in and near the heart after intravenous injection of a radiopharmaceutical. Sequential images are recorded with a scintillation camera.

Radiopaque: impenetrable by X-rays or any other form of radiation.

Radiopharmaceutical: a radioactive preparation that is injected or given by mouth in certain diagnostic or treatment procedures.

Radiosensitive: capable of being damaged or destroyed by radiation, as a tumor, cell, or tissue.

Rapid plasma reagin test: a blood test to detect syphilis.

Normal value in plasma: negative

Rapid surfactant test: an amniotic fluid test to determine fetal lung maturity.

Normal values in AF: a complete ring of bubbles persisting 15 minutes at 1:1 dilution only

Receptors: cellular surface structures that combine with antigen or other substances and thereby acquire new properties.

Recurrent infection: repeat bouts of the same type of infection in the same person.

Red blood cell count: a count of the number of red blood cells in a specimen of whole blood.

Normal values in whole blood: males—4.6-6.2 million/mm^3; females—4.2-5.4 million/mm^3

Reducing substances, total: a test performed on urine to measure the levels of glucose and other natural sugars.

Normal values in urine after 24-hour collection: total sugars—250 mg; glucose—130 mg

Refractive index: a measurement of the total solids in a solution, done by detecting the change in the pathways of light going through the solution.

Remission: a period of time during which there is no evidence of a previously existing disease.

Renal angiography: X-ray studies of the blood vessels surrounding the kidneys, after injection of contrast medium.

Renal arteriography: X-ray studies of the renal artery and related blood vessels, after injection of contrast medium.

Renal scan: a scan of the kidneys for size, shape, and exact location, to diagnose a tumor or other abnormalities; done after intravenous injection of a radioactive substance.

Renin test: *see* Plasma renin activity.

Resident bacteria: bacteria usually found living in a given body area.

Residual volume: the amount of air retained in the lungs after exhaling.

Reticulocyte: a type of red blood cell comprising about 1% of the red cells in the bloodstream.

Reticulocyte count: a test to determine the number of reticulocytes in a specimen of whole blood, a measure of bone marrow activity; decreased in hemolytic (blood cell destroying) disease; elevated after hemorrhage, or while recovering from anemia.

Normal values in whole blood: 25,000-75,000 cells/microliter

Retrograde pyelogram: radiographic record of the kidneys and urinary tract, using an instrument inserted in the bladder to inject the contrast medium directly into the urinary tract.

Rheumatoid factor: a blood factor present in rheumatoid arthritis and various infectious diseases.

Normal values in serum: sensitized sheep cell method—titer of less than 1:160; latex fixation method—titer of less than 1:80; bentonite particles method—titer of less than 1:32

Rh factor: a blood factor present in most, but not all people. An Rh-negative person can develop antibodies to the Rh factor if exposed to it through blood transfusion or pregnancy. An Rh-positive infant of a woman with Rh antibodies may be born with a serious blood disease. Administration of an immune human globulin (RhoGAM) to an Rh-negative mother within 72 hours of giving birth to an Rh-positive infant will prevent the development of antibodies and protect her future pregnancies.

Ribonucleic acid: one of two types of nucleic acids that transmit hereditary factors.

Rickettsiae: tiny microorganisms that live in cells and are considered somewhere between bacteria and viruses in structure.

Roentgen: a unit of measure; the amount of radiation that produces 1 electrostatic unit of electricity in 1 cubic centimeter of air.

Roentgen equivalent, man: a unit that measures the biologic effect of radiation on the human body.

Rollover test: test during pregnancy for susceptibility to toxemia of pregnancy—a serious high blood pressure condition of unknown origin.

Normal value in the pregnant woman: As her position is changed from lying on the left side to lying on the back, there is no change or elevation of blood pressure.

Rubacell: a blood test done to determine whether a child or adult has had rubella (German measles), to screen for immunity to rubella, and to determine whether a child has a congenital rubella infection.

S

Salicylate: a salt of salicylic acid present in blood during treatment with aspirin or aspirin-like drugs.

Normal values in serum: negative;
therapeutic level—20-25 mg/dl

Saprophyte: an organism that feeds on dead organic matter.

Schick test: a skin test to detect susceptibility or exposure to diphtheria.

Schiller test: a test for abnormalities of the cervix. Iodine is applied to distinguish normal areas, which accept the stain, and abnormal areas, which don't.

Schilling test: a test of vitamin B_{12} blood levels, in which radioactive B_{12} is given orally and measured in 24-hour urine. An abnormal level may be the cause of anemia or other disease conditions.

Normal values in urine: 8-40% of radioactive B_{12} previously ingested

---

Scintiscan: a map of the distribution in the body, or in a body part, of a radioactive compound (radiopharmaceutical) given previously; the emitted rays are printed on photographic film.

Secondary infection: a new infection in a person who already has an infection.

Sedimentation: settling of solid material in blood or other fluid to the bottom of a container.

Sedimentation rate: *see under* Erythrocyte.

Seminal fluid, liquefaction: a test of the duration of the liquefaction process in seminal fluid. If delayed, it may indicate abnormalities such as congenital absence of certain internal sexual organs.

Normal values: complete within 20 minutes

Seminal fluid, morphology: a test of the percentage of normally formed spermatozoa in the seminal fluid; important in fertility studies.

Normal values: more than 70% normal, mature sperm

Seminal fluid, motility: a test of the percentage of normally motile spermatozoa in the seminal fluid; important in fertility studies.

Normal values: more than 60% of sperm motile

Seminal fluid, pH: the degree of alkalinity or acidity of seminal fluid; important in fertility studies and diagnostic evaluations of the internal sexual organs.

Normal values: more than 7.0 (average: 7.7)

Seminal fluid, sperm count: a test of the quantity of sperm in the seminal fluid; important in fertility studies.

Normal values: 60-150 million/ml (average: 100 million)

Seminal fluid, volume: a test of the amount of seminal fluid produced in an ejaculation.

Normal values: 1.5-5.0 ml

Sepsis: poisoning of body cells by infectious organisms or by the toxic substances they produce.

Septicemia: poisoning of the bloodstream by infectious organisms or the toxins they produce.

Sequential multiple analysis (SMA-6, SMA-12, SMA-18): the biochemical examination of 6, 12, or 18 blood constituents via a multichannel laboratory apparatus.

Serosanguineous fluid: blood and tissue fluids that drain from a wound.

Serotonin, *see* 5-Hydroxytryptamine.

Serum: the fluid portion of blood that remains after the blood has clotted.

Serum glutamic-oxaloacetic transaminase: *see* Transaminases

Sialography: X-ray studies of the parotid and submaxillary glands (situated below and behind the jawbones) after injection of contrast medium.

Sigmoidoscopy: internal examination of the sigmoid (lowest portion of large bowel) with a scope, to detect abnormalities such as polyps or tumors.

Simplate bleeding time test: a blood test to determine the ability of the platelets to form a plug—the first step in clotting when platelets are exposed to air. Delay in forming the plug may be due to platelet deficiency or to a drug, such as aspirin.

Normal values in fresh, standard-size forearm incision: 2-8 minutes

SMA: *see* Sequential multiple analysis.

Smear: a thin layer of tissue or fluid spread on a glass slide for microscopic examination.

Sodium (in blood): a normal blood constituent, essential in transmitting nerve impulses, and in maintaining water metabolism and acid/base balance.

Normal values in plasma: 136-142 mEq/liter

Sodium (in sweat): the level of sodium in sweat; elevated in fibrocystic disease.

Normal values in sweat: 10-80 mEq/liter

Sodium (in urine): a normal constituent of urine, measured to check adrenal function, kidney function, acid/base balance, and other conditions.

Normal values in urine after 24-hour collection:
80-180 mEq

Specific gravity: the concentration of solutes in a urine specimen compared with a standard specimen; may be altered by disease and other factors.

Normal values with normal fluid intake: 1.016-1.022

Specimen: a sample of body tissue or fluid.

Spectrophotometry: *see under* Atomic.

Spinal fluid, *see* Cerebrospinal fluid.

Spinal tap: removal of fluid from the spinal canal by means of a needle and syringe.

Spleen scan: a scan of the spleen after injection of radioactive red blood cells, done to detect a tumor, injury, or other abnormality.

Splenoportography: X-ray studies of the spleen, liver, and nearby blood vessels, after injection of contrast medium into the spleen.

Spore: the reproductive element of fungi and certain bacteria.

Sputum: a mixture of lung and tracheobronchial secretions that are coughed up and may be examined for harmful microorganisms.

Sputum culture: incubation of a sample of sputum in nutrient material to determine the growth and type of infection-causing microorganisms.

Stain: a dye used to color bacteria or tissues to make them visible for examination under the microscope.

Staphylococcus: a type of disease-causing bacteria that grow in the form of clusters resembling grapes. Common species include Staph aureus, Staph epidermidis, and Staph saprophyticus.

Stereotaxic neuroradiography: an X-ray procedure generally done in the operating room during neurosurgery, that guides the insertion of a needle into a desired location in the brain.

Sterile: free of microorganisms.

Steroid hormones: the sex hormones and adrenal cortical hormones.

Stool culture: incubation of a sample of feces in nutrient material to determine growth and types of infection-causing microorganisms.

Streptococcal MG agglutinin test: a test for pneumonia or other pulmonary infections caused by certain streptococcus strains.

Normal values in serum: titer of less than 1:20

Streptococcus: a type of disease-causing bacteria that grow in the form of chains. Common species include Strep pneumoniae and Strep pyogenes.

Streptolysins O and S: the poisonous substances produced by certain forms of streptococci known as beta hemolytic because they can destroy blood cells.

Stress electrocardiogram: an ECG tracing that is made while the patient exercises on a treadmill or stationary bicycle, to evaluate heart muscle function.

Normal values while exercising: no change in ECG, except for an increase in heart rate

Sulfhemoglobin: a substance not normally present in the blood, but found in patients who have taken certain drugs in excess, or in cases of hydrogen sulfide poisoning.

Normal value in whole blood: negative

Sulfonamides: a class of bacteriostatic medications used to treat infection.

Normal value in serum or whole blood: negative

Superinfection: growth of certain harmful organisms normally kept in check by other organisms that are temporarily being destroyed by an antibiotic medication.

Surgical sponge radiography: X-ray studies to locate a surgical sponge in the operative area during, or just after, surgery.

Susceptibility: the state of being receptive to infection or disease.

Syndrome: a set of symptoms that tend to appear together.

Synovial fluid: viscid fluid secreted by the membrane that lines a joint cavity.

Synovial fluid-blood glucose difference: difference in glucose levels between blood and synovial fluid, which may be increased in arthritis and certain other conditions.

Normal difference: less than 10 mg/dl

Synovial fluid, differential cell count: a test in which cells are differentiated and counted to detect inflammation or infection.

Normal values: granulocytes constitute fewer than 25% of nucleated cells

Synovial fluid, fibrin clot: a clot present during inflammation or infection.

Normal value: negative

Synovial fluid, mucin clot: clot whose quality may be fair to poor in inflammation or infection.

Normal value: abundant

Synovial fluid, nucleated cell count: a count elevated in inflammatory or infectious conditions, as well as after hemorrhage.

Normal values: fewer than 200 cells/microliter

Synovial fluid, viscosity: property that may be decreased in inflammatory or septic conditions.

Normal value: high

Synovial fluid, volume: the amount of synovial fluid in a joint, which may be increased in trauma or other abnormal conditions.

Normal values: less than 3.5 ml

T

Tartrazine sensitivity: sensitivity to tartrazine, a substance found in some foods (e.g., sweet potatoes) and used as a color additive in foods and drugs.

Terminal disinfection: a method of removing disease-causing organisms and their toxins from a room previously occupied by a patient who had an infectious disease.

Terminal infection: an infection that causes death.

Testosterone: male hormone present in blood; important in diagnosing poor function of the testes (decreased level) and testicular cancer (increased level).

Normal values in serum or plasma:
males—400-1,200 ng/dl; females—30-120 ng/dl

Theophylline: a medication used to treat asthma; monitored in the blood to maintain levels adequate to prevent or stop respiratory problems, but not high enough to cause toxic reactions.

Therapeutic levels: 40-100 mcg/ml of whole blood

Thermography: measurement of temperature variations in soft tissues; a useful technique for detecting various abnormalities.

Thoracentesis: removal of fluid from inside the chest wall with a syringe and needle, for diagnostic or treatment purposes.

Throat culture: incubation of a sample of throat secretions in nutrient material, to determine the presence and type of infection-causing microorganisms.

Thromboplastin generation time: the time it takes whole blood to generate thromboplastin, a coagulation factor. Deficient thromboplastin generation causes bleeding problems.

Normal values in whole blood: 12 seconds or less (100%)

Thymol flocculation (turbidity): a blood test to determine functional capacity of the liver; performed by mixing a serum sample with thymol. Increased turbidity (cloudiness) indicates liver disease such as hepatitis.

Normal values in serum: 0-5 turbidity units

Thyroid antibodies: antibodies present in various diseases, such as thyroid disease, allergic disorders, and pernicious anemia.

Normal values in serum: antithyroglobulin antibody—titer of less than 1:32; antithyroid microsomal antibody—titer of less than 1:56

Thyroid hormone tests (triiodothyronine, T_3; thyroxine, T_4; thyroxine-binding globulin, TBG): tests done to determine the levels of thyroid hormones for diagnosing various thyroid disorders.

Normal values in serum expressed as iodine:
T_4 (by column)—3.2-7.2 mcg/dl; T_4 (by competitive binding)—3.9-7.7 mcg/dl; free T_4—0.6-1.5 ng/dl

Normal values in serum expressed as thyroxine:
T_4 (by column)—5-11 mcg/dl; T_4 (by competitive binding)—6-11.8 mcg/dl; free T_4—0.9-2.3 ng/dl;
T_3 (resin uptake)—25-38% relative uptake;
TBG—10-26 mcg/dl

Thyroid microsomal antibody: an antibody to thyroid present when the patient has an autoimmune reaction that originates in the thyroid gland (*see* Thyroid antibodies).

Thyroid scan: an organ imaging procedure done after injecting a radioactive substance into a vein, to determine the thyroid's size, shape, location, and function, or any abnormality such as cancer.

Thyroid stimulation test: a procedure in which the patient is given thyroid-stimulating hormone (TSH), a secretion of the pituitary gland. Its effects on the thyroid are then observed, to determine whether thyroid problems are due to pituitary or thyroid dysfunction.

Thyroid ^{131}I uptake: a test for thyroid disorders; the thyroid's absorption of oral or intravenous radioactive iodine is measured with a scintillation counter at 1, 6, or 24 hours after ingestion.

Normal values: 9-19% in 1 hour; 7.5-25% in 6 hours; 10-50% in 24 hours

Thyroxine: a thyroid hormone measured in venous blood; elevated in hyperthyroidism and decreased in hypothyroidism. (*See* Thyroid hormone tests.)

Timed forced expiratory volume: a measurement of lung capacity.

Normal values: 80% air exhaled in first second and 95% air exhaled by the third second

Tissue: an accumulation of cells that forms an identifiable structure, such as skin.

Tissue culture: the process of growing cells outside the body for various diagnostic or research purposes.

Titer: the strength, or concentration, of a substance in fluid, such as the lowest dilution of serum at which antibody is still present.

Tomography: a special X-ray technique that visualizes layers of tissues.

Tonometry: the use of an instrument (tonometer) to measure the fluid pressure inside the eyeball, mainly to test for glaucoma, a condition in which fluid pressure is elevated.

Total iron-binding capacity: *see* Iron-binding capacity.

Normal values: 200-400 mcg/dl

Total lung capacity: *see* Total lung volume.

Total lung volume: the size of the lungs and their dead space, in liters, measured by having the patient rebreathe a gas such as helium.

Toxemia: a condition in which toxins produced by bacteria poison the bloodstream, usually as a result of an overwhelming infection.

Toxin: a poisonous metabolic product of living organisms, usually of disease-causing microorganisms such as bacteria.

Toxoid: a product prepared from bacterial toxins that has been treated so it is no longer toxic but can still stimulate the production of antitoxin against bacterial infections such as diphtheria or tetanus. It is therefore a useful agent in immunization.

Toxoplasma antibodies: antibodies to the parasite Toxoplasma gondii, which causes toxoplasmosis, an infectious disease often spread via cat feces.

Normal values in serum: titer of less than 1:4

Transaminases: the enzymes serum glutamic-oxaloacetic transaminase (SGOT, also known as aspartate aminotransferase) and serum glutamic-pyruvic transaminase (SGPT, also known as alanine aminotransferase). Blood levels of these enzymes are measured to diagnose liver and heart disease.

Normal values in serum: SGOT—8-33 units/ml;
SGPT—1-36 units/ml

Transferrin: an iron-binding protein in the blood; levels are increased in iron deficiency and decreased in inflammatory conditions and liver disease.

Normal values in whole blood: 300-359 mg/dl

Transfusion: the injection of fluid, blood, or blood components into a vein to counteract depletion of fluid, blood, or blood components.

Trichina (Trichinella) agglutinin test: a test performed to detect the presence of trichinosis, a disease contracted by persons who eat undercooked, infected pork or beef.

Normal values in serum: negative

Triglycerides: fatty substances measured in the blood. They may be elevated in heart and blood vessel diseases.

Normal values in serum: 10-190 mg/dl

Triiodothyronine (T_3) resin uptake: incorporation of radioactive T_3 and synthetic resin particles by serum, tested to determine whether the patient has hyperthyroidism or hypothyroidism.

Trypsin activity test: a test done on feces for the presence of trypsin; done to diagnose fibrocystic disease of the pancreas, respiratory system, sweat glands, or other organ systems.

Normal values in random, fresh feces: trypsin 2+ to 4+

Tuberculin: a substance derived from tubercle bacilli (tuberculosis-causing organisms), used to diagnose tuberculosis or exposure to the disease.

Tuberculin test: a skin test using tuberculin, to detect susceptibility or exposure to tuberculosis.

Tularemia agglutinin test: a test to determine the presence of tularemia, an infectious disease spread through contact with infected rabbits.

Normal values in serum: titer of less than 1:80

Tuning-fork tests: tests in which a tuning fork is used to measure hearing function and bone-conduction sensitivity in various neurologic (nervous-system) examinations.

Turbidimetry: measurement of the transmission of light through a suspension, used to determine the presence of protein in urine, spinal fluid, or plasma, and in the quantitation of bacteria and antigen-antibody complexes.

Tympanometry: a test to determine whether allergy or infection is interfering with adequate functioning of the eardrum. Varying tones are administered to the outer ear canal, and the pressure response within the ear is recorded on a graph.

Typhoid agglutinin test: a test on serum to diagnose the presence of typhoid fever.

Normal values: O—titer of less than 1:80;
H—titer of less than 1:80

Typing: classifying blood, tissues, cells, disease-causing organisms, and other materials so they can be compared with standards.

U

Ultrasound: high-frequency sound waves used to project images of various parts of the body. A transducer produces the ultrasound and catches the response, which is displayed on an oscilloscope.

Unsaturated vitamin B_{12} binding capacity: a test that measures the ability of vitamin B_{12} to bind with a protein called intrinsic factor in the stomach, prior to absorption in the bowel.

Normal values in serum: 1-2 ng/ml of free vitamin B_{12}

Urea clearance: the amount of urea filtered and removed from the blood by the kidneys within a given period of time.

Normal values in serum and urine: maximum clearance—64-99 ml/minute; standard clearance—41-65 ml/minute, or more than 75% of normal clearance

---

Urea nitrogen (in blood): a nitrogen fraction elevated in the serum of patients with certain kidney and other diseases.

Normal values in serum: 10-20 mg/dl

Urea nitrogen (in urine): a nitrogen fraction elevated in the urine in certain kidney and other diseases.

Normal values in urine after 24-hour collection: 6-17 gm

Uric acid: substance elevated in the serum in various diseases such as gout, and decreased if the patient is taking anticoagulants or antiworm medicine.

Normal values: males—2.1-7.8 mg/dl; females—2.0-6.4 mg/dl

Urinary creatinine clearance: *see* Creatinine.

Urine specimen, 24-hour: all the urine voided in a 24-hour period; necessary for certain urine tests, such as the creatinine clearance test.

Urobilinogen (in feces): a bilirubin metabolism product found in the feces; increased in certain types of blood diseases and decreased in certain liver, gallbladder, and related diseases.

Normal values: qualitative, random specimen—positive; quantitative, in 24-hour specimen—40-200 mg

Urobilinogen, urinary: a bilirubin metabolism product found in urine; increased in certain diseases causing red blood cell destruction.

Normal values in urine: after 2 hours—0.3-1.0 Ehrlich unit; after 24 hours—0.05-2.5 mg (0.5-4.0 Ehrlich units)

Uroporphyrins: substances present in the urine in congenital or metabolic disease, such as porphyria.

Normal values in urine: qualitative, random specimen—absent; quantitative, 24-hour specimen—10-30 mcg

V

Vaccination: introduction of an antibody-stimulating substance (antigen) into the body.

Vaccine: a substance made from disease-causing material that has been modified so it will not cause disease when introduced into the body, but will stimulate the formation of antibodies to that disease.

Vanillylmandelic acid: *see* 3-Methoxy-4-hydroxymandelic acid.

Vector: a carrier of disease-causing microorganisms from one host to another (examples: a fly, louse, or mosquito).

Vectorcardiogram, spatial: a three-dimensional electrocardiogram that shows electrical activity in the heart muscle projected on three coordinates simultaneously, as well as muscle contraction and relaxation.

Vein scan: scanning procedure performed after intravenous injection of a radiopharmaceutical, to detect blood clots or inflammation.

Venereal: caused or spread by sexual contact.

Venereal Disease Research Laboratory test: a blood test for syphilis.

Normal values in serum: nonreactive

Venography: a radiographic procedure that shows the internal structures of veins after the patient receives an injection of contrast medium.

Venous impedance plethysmography: a procedure that measures blood flow through a vein to detect the presence of a clot.

Ventilation scan (lung scan): procedure in which the patient breathes in radioactive gas and the lungs are scanned for areas that don't receive air, or other abnormalities.

Ventriculography: X-ray studies of the ventricles of the brain, involving the insertion of needles to withdraw fluid and inject air or gas.

Viremia: a viral infection of the blood.

Virulence: the capacity of a given organism or group of organisms to produce disease of various degrees of severity.

Virus: a minute organism that lives in cells and can cause disease.

Virus-neutralizing antibodies: antibodies that render a virus harmless.

Viscosity: glue-like or sticky property of a semiliquid substance.

Normal values in whole blood: 1.4-1.8 times that of water

Vital capacity: lung volume; measured as the patient breathes in, then exhales as much air as possible.

Normal values: about 4-6 liters/exhalation

Vitamin A (retinol): a fat-soluble vitamin present in inadequate amounts in poor nutrition and in certain other conditions, such as use of oral contraceptives or excessive consumption of mineral oil.

Normal values in serum: 30-60 mcg/dl

Vitamin A tolerance: a test of the body's capacity to react to a given dose of vitamin A. Failure of serum levels to rise to normal within 4-5 hours indicates inadequate intestinal fat absorption.

Normal values in serum (after giving 5,000 U Vit A/kg in oil): fasting—15-60 mcg/dl; after 3 or 6 hours—200-600 mcg/dl; after 24 hours—fasting level or slightly higher

Vitamin B_1 (thiamine): a vitamin present in inadequate amounts in poor nutrition, alcoholism, and other conditions.

Normal values in whole blood: 1.5-4 mcg/dl

Normal values in urine: 25-75 mcg/dl

Vitamin B_2 (riboflavin): a vitamin whose deficiency may cause eye and skin problems as well as abnormal states of the blood and nervous system.

Normal values in blood: over 15 mcg/dl of red blood cells

Normal values in 6-hour urine: 30-60 mcg

Vitamin B_3 (niacin): a vitamin whose deficiency may cause skin, nervous-system, and intestinal problems. Deficiency may be caused by alcoholism.

Normal values in 6-hour urine: 0.6-1.5 mg

Vitamin B_6 (pyridoxine): a vitamin whose deficiency may cause eye, skin, and nervous-system problems.

Normal values in urine after 24-hour collection: 35-55 mcg

Vitamin B_{12} (cyanocobalamin) test, blood: a test of the body's ability to absorb and utilize vitamin B_{12}; decreased in pernicious anemia, after surgical removal of the stomach, in alcoholism, gastrointestinal infection, and various other conditions.

Normal values in serum: males—200-800 pg/ml; females—100-650 pg/ml

---

Vitamin B_{12} (cyanocobalamin) test, urine: a test to detect deficiency of this vitamin, which can cause anemia, inadequate growth of tissues, and poor function of the nervous system.

Normal values: 8-40% of the radioactive vitamin B_{12} previously ingested by mouth

Vitamin C (ascorbic acid): a vitamin whose deficiency may cause skin, gum, and hair problems, and interfere with tooth and bone development.

Normal values in plasma: 0.6-2.0 mg/dl

Normal values in urine after 24-hour collection: more than 50 mg

Vitamin D, alkaline phosphatase test: a test to detect vitamin D deficiency, which may cause rickets, softening of the bones (osteomalacia), and tooth decay.

Normal alkaline phosphatase levels in serum:
adults—2-4.5 Bodansky units/dl;
children—5-15 Bodansky units/dl

Vitamin E (tocopherol): a vitamin whose deficiency may cause anemia and infertility.

Normal value in plasma: 0.5 mg/dl

Vitamin K: a vitamin whose deficiency may cause inadequate clotting of the blood.

Normal values in plasma: 12-14 seconds (prothrombin time)

Vollmer test: a patch (skin) test to determine the presence of tuberculosis or previous exposure to the disease.

Volume, total: the total amount of urine excreted in a 24-hour period; measured to assess kidney function.

Normal values: 600-1,600 ml/24 hours

W

Weil-Felix test (Proteus OX-2, OX-K, and OX-19 agglutinins): a test to determine the presence of typhus and other rickettsial diseases.

Normal values in serum: 4-fold rise in titer between acute and convalescent sera

---

White blood cell count: a count of the white blood cells in a specimen of whole blood.

Normal values in whole blood: 4,500-11,000/mm^3

White blood count, differential: a test done on blood to determine the types and proportions of the different types of white blood cells in a specimen of whole blood.

Normal values in whole blood (mean and range):
segmented neutrophils: 56%; 1-7 ml
bands: 3%; 0-700 μl
eosinophils: 2.7%; 0-450 μl
basophils: 0.3%; 0-200 μl
lymphocytes: 34%; 1-4.8 ml
monocytes: 4%; 0-800 μl

Wound culture: a culture done on a sample of wound drainage to determine the presence of disease-causing organisms.

X

Xanthochromia, cerebrospinal fluid test: a test to determine whether yellow color—due to breakdown of red blood cells—is present in the CSF, which may indicate hemorrhage, jaundice, very high protein levels, or a traumatic spinal tap.

Normal value in CSF: negative

X-rays (Roentgen rays): rays emitted by special equipment that penetrate the body to a calculated depth for diagnostic or treatment purposes.

Xylose absorption test: a test done to determine the rate of absorption of xylose, a wood sugar, into blood. Absorption is impaired in certain disorders of fat absorption.

Normal values in serum: 25-40 mg/dl between 1 and 2 hours; in malabsorption, maximum approximately 10 mg/dl

---

Z

Zinc (in blood): the level of zinc in the serum, elevated in zinc poisoning and some other conditions.

Normal values: 50-150 mcg/dl

Zinc (in urine): the level of zinc in the urine, elevated in zinc poisoning and some other conditions.

Normal values in urine after 24-hour collection:
0.15-1.2 mg (trace)

Zinc sulfate turbidity test: a test done to determine the gamma globulin concentration in blood; increased in infection, allergy, and autoimmune illnesses, and decreased in some leukemias, cancers, and hypoimmune conditions.

Normal values in serum: less than 12 units

Zonography: a technique of tissue-layer X-ray study that blurs all tissue layers above and below the layer needed for the study.

Zoonosis: disease found in animals that is transmissible to humans.

Bibliography

Garb, Solomon, M.D. *Laboratory Tests in Common Use*. New York: Springer Publishing Co., 1976.

Widmann, Frances K., M.D. *Clinical Interpretation of Laboratory Tests*. Philadelphia: F.A. Davis Co., 1979.

Davidsohn, Israel, M.D., and Henry, John B., M.D., eds. *Clinical Diagnosis by Laboratory Methods,* Todd-Sanford. Philadelphia: W.B. Saunders Co., 1974.

Collins, R. Douglas, M.D. *Illustrated Manual of Laboratory Diagnosis*. Philadelphia: J.B. Lippincott Co., 1975.

Berkow, Robert, M.D., ed., and Talbott, John H., M.D., consulting ed. *Merck Manual of Diagnosis and Therapy,* 13th ed. Rahway, N.J.: Merck and Co., Inc., 1977.

Fischbach, Frances T., R.N. *A Manual of Laboratory Diagnostic Tests*. Philadelphia: J.B. Lippincott Co., 1980.

Conte, Sylvester B., and Kemme, Douglas H. *Positioning and Technique Handbook for Radiologic Technologists*. St. Louis: C.V. Mosby Co., 1978.

Physicians' Desk Reference for Radiology and Nuclear Medicine, 1979/80 ed. Oradell, N.J.: Medical Economics Co., 1979.

Clinical Laboratory Reference, Medical Laboratory Observer, 7th ed. Oradell, N.J.: Medical Economics Co., 1980.

Smith, Alice L. *Microbiology and Pathology,* 12th ed. St. Louis: C.V. Mosby Co., 1980.